THE FUTURE OF MEDICAL JOURNALS:

IN COMMEMORATION OF 150 YEARS OF THE *BRITISH MEDICAL JOURNAL*

THE FUTURE OF MEDICAL JOURNALS:

IN COMMEMORATION OF 150 YEARS OF THE *BRITISH MEDICAL JOURNAL*

Edited by

Stephen P Lock

editor, *British Medical Journal*, 1975–91

Published by the British Medical Journal
Tavistock Square, London WC1H 9JR

First edition 1991

ISBN 0 7279 0312 8

Made and printed in England by
Latimer Trend & Company Ltd, Plymouth

Contents

III THE COMMUNICATION OF CLINICAL INFORMATION

IV THE TECHNOLOGIES OF INFORMATION

V THE FUTURE

Introduction

STEPHEN LOCK

No one has yet found an ideal way of publishing the outcome of discussions at scientific seminars. Readers of the proceedings concentrate on the formal papers, skipping the unstructured questions and comments. No doubt a creative and selective editor may occasionally distill a taut dialogue out of myriad separate strands and exclude the inevitable irrelevancies and side issues. The volumes of Ciba Foundation Symposia show what may be achieved with a broad subject and lots of detail. Attempting this for discussions where these conditions are not present, however, is likely to be disappointing for all concerned.

Given these provisos, I abandoned the idea of publishing the transcripts of the discussions at the meeting on the future of biomedical journals. To be sure, the seminar itself was first class. The participants included many of the editors of our principal general medical journals on both sides of the Atlantic, an information scientist, a sociologist, and epidemiologists, and they produced stimulating papers full of new ideas and insights. The discussions were free and prolonged, but there were really only two major themes—the scientific quality of medical journals and the relevance of their content to clinicians. It will help the reader more, I believe, if I devote my Introduction to considering and summarising those two topics.

The first scientific journal was published in 1665, establishing a pattern that soon led to a rapid and sustained growth of further publications. For most of the 330 years since the appearance of the *Journal de Scavans* and the *Philosophical Transactions of the Royal Society* growth was maintained at around 7% a year; recently the rate of increase has slowed slightly but there is no sign of any substantial diminution in the growth of new journals. Derek de Solla Price, who first proposed this pattern, also showed the logic behind it. New disciplines emerge every 10 years and need to have

1

their own specialty journals, where (initially at least) the authorship is the same as the readership.[1] Thus, Franklin said at the Leeds Castle seminar, given the right subdiscipline, publishers still find it economic to introduce new journals with a circulation of only 300–400.

The health of these scientific biomedical journals is, however, more apparent than real. For, as speaker after speaker emphasised, the journals are serving the community poorly. Many articles are neither read nor cited; indeed, many articles are poor. In general, medical journals seem to be of little practical help to clinicians facing problems at the bedside. Nor are some of the general journals offering any effective leadership on contemporary issues such as healthcare policy, unemployment, and the population explosion. And underlying these worries was yet another: that scientific articles have been hijacked away from their primary role of communicating scientific discovery to one of demonstrating academic activity. No more are grant giving bodies basing awards on the quality of scientific research; the emphasis has switched to quantity.

With such a formidable indictment we must consider some of the details of the charges. Firstly, how many published articles do go ignored and unread? The evidence is depressing. In Warren's study of 10 000 references on schistosomiasis, for example, 50 experts did not mention 70% of the articles even once and only 400 articles came up on more than six occasions. Similarly, Haynes found that in an average literature search 15% of the references are relevant and valid but that these come up at random. Library use studies have shown that in the course of a year at least half the journals on the shelves are never looked at at all.

Once articles can be ordered from on line full text services, such as ADONIS, the small proportion of articles scientists actually read is likely to be emphasised even further. Moreover, a recent citation study from the Institute for Scientific Information, published three months after the seminar was held, has not only confirmed these findings for biomedicine but also shown how the latter compares with other disciplines.[2] Analysis showed that 55% of the papers the Institute covers did not receive a single citation in the five years after they appeared (1984–8). The proportions varied from one discipline to another: with 46·4% of articles uncited, medicine fell just below the average of 47·4% for the 'hard' sciences (all disciplines excluding social science, which had an uncited average of 74·7%). Outside biomedicine there were dramatic variations: at one end of the scale, in atomic, molecular, and chemical physics, only 9·2% of articles were uncited. By contrast, 99·9% of those about theatre and 98·2% about religion received no citations and presumably were little read.

Similar good evidence exists that in medicine many articles are (scientifically) seriously flawed or contain too little information for the discerning reader even when this might have been available to the authors. Most work in the analysis of this problem has been done on the statistical handling of data.[3] Defects in the statistics can sometimes be corrected by thorough peer review,[4] but Williamson and his colleagues have also documented the general inadequacy of a large number of articles.[5] They reviewed the 28 most valid assessments of the scientific adequacy of study design, data, statistical references, and documentation in over 4200 research reports. In reports published before 1970 a median of 23% of 2063 research reports met the reviewers' criteria; in those published after 1970 the median was only 6% in 2172 reports. Moreover, when design, analysis, and documentation were assessed concurrently, the proportion of articles meeting the criteria often dropped to under 1%. Given that these were usually assessments of articles in the leading medical journals, they commented that the quality of the entire medical literature is likely to be much worse.

For the past 20 years repeated efforts have been made to encourage authors to improve the reporting and analysis of their results, but there is no evidence that this has happened. Nor do these criticisms apply only to original articles. In review articles, Chalmers emphasised, the rules of science are often disregarded, with no definition of material and methods or the rules for including or excluding studies, no ensuring that the samples were representative of the available evidence, and no controls for bias or the use of proper statistical techniques.

Even if the scientific presentations of research studies could be improved, however, many clinicians would continue to complain that their content is rarely relevant to the real world of practical medicine. From a study of five journals in internal medicine, seven general journals, and nine major specialty journals Haynes pointed out that a general internist would have to read 10, 20, and 25 articles, respectively, to discover one article giving information about a specific beneficial effect. Almost two fifths of the practitioners and a third of the 'opinion leaders' in Williamson's survey found great difficulties in sorting out irrelevant material in published articles.

Even more depressing, given these data, is that when an article does appear reporting an advance in clinical medicine many years pass before there is any observable change in practice. For example, several years elapsed between the description of the beneficial effects of angiotensin converting enzyme inhibitors in cardiac failure and their general use by clinicians. A published survey by Williamson and his colleagues has produced similar findings.[6] Asked about their use of six recent clinical advances (such as the measurement of glycated haemoglobin as an aid to controlling diabetes), between one fifth and one half of doctors were not aware of the techniques or were not using them.

The whole discussion at the seminar, Huth concluded, underscored the strong care for research into what readers need; there are many ex cathedra statements about what clinicians ought to be reading, yet they say that their prime need is for 'ready knowledge'—Riis's term for synoptic information, which at present they get largely from textbooks and lectures.

As a result of all these factors, the seminar heard, doctors are turning increasingly to the 'throwaway' journals, which present crisp messages attractively. Yet these are primarily motivated by commercial considerations; the articles may be dangerously simplistic in their conclusions, and these are not subjected to editorial per review.

In the Third World the state of affairs is even worse. There journals are mostly of indifferent physical quality, contain poor science, come out late (many listed do not appear at all), and are less read than foreign journals—where most of the country's top scientists publish their best work. Articles tend to be accepted without peer review and published in order of receipt.

Next, in Richard Smith's view particularly, general biomedical journals are failing in their larger duty to society by abrogating any leadership role. They ignore the problems of the larger world, such as pollution, undernutrition, and the population explosion. Medical journals (particularly the general ones) should have an enduring purpose to raise the level of debate on medicine and health. A prime aim should be to improve patient care, educating doctors about literacy, their daily tasks, and social and political issues such as health economics, which had not even been heard of 25 years ago. And where they had failed in particular was in supplying leadership about how health care systems should develop; mostly they had reacted to proposals made by others rather than making proposals of their own. Finally, if this accusation could be levelled at general journals then another could be made against the specialist clinical ones—which in Booth's opinion had become dominated by clinicians in the sponsoring societies. As a result, editors came under heavy pressure to publish poor case series, with only minimal clinical relevance, and ignored important developments in basic science and epidemiology. The vital interface between clinical medicine and other disciplines had been lost, yet the advances in molecular biology had changed the direction of scientific progress: it was now centripetal rather than centrifugal. Scientists working in molecular biology might be dermatologists one month and, that question answered, haematologists the next.

It would be wrong, however, to imply that the whole flavour of the seminar was negative. Having analysed the deficiences, the participants turned to proposals for correcting them. And it was then that the group split into two factions—taking up positions similar to those of the two great 17th century philosophers Thomas Hobbes and John Locke. The 'Hobbesians' wanted to introduce devices such as guidelines, checklists, and structured abstracts to get authors to improve the scientific rigour of articles (and referees to monitor whether key features were present). By contrast, the Lockeians would rely on a powerful and knowledgeable medical editor and his advisers to achieve the same ends. Stringent rules, the Lockeians argued, might stifle creativity and divert a referee's attention away from an article's message—nor could a single check-list be applied to the wide variety of articles journals received. Yet, the Hobbesians riposted, devices such as structured abstracts had been developed specifically for articles most relevant for clinicians, dealing with diagnosis, treatment, prognosis, causation, quality of care, and health economics. And using checklists would improve those articles which fail to mention important detail that is available.

As a Hobbesian myself, I have to be careful in presenting a balanced argument, and the plain fact is that most editors are not totally polarised in one direction or another—they have mixed feelings and, to quote Joseph Stalin about the poet Anna Akhmatova, are 'half nun, half whore.' They have after all agreed about various constraints on authors in the interests of improving the quality of articles—in particular, the guidelines produced by the Vancouver group on reference style, retraction of duplicate publication, and definition of authorship, and these recommendations seem likely to continue. And, for example, ensuring that both editors and referees get a better training in methodology won universal support. In Riis's view, this aspect is 'tainted' in 70–80% of articles and the discussion sections in articles rarely include a proper critique of the methods used. Another suggestion that was favoured was to ask referees to target key issues rather than slavishly completing a checklist.

There was also consensus that editors needed to make their journals much more attractive to readers, ensuring that the articles are as readable as possible. But, though clinicians are not very good at distinguishing which articles tell them useful validated information, on which they should act from preliminary observations, many of the discussants drew the line at the suggestion for 'pink' pages. Under this the articles would be classified into different sections—for example, definite clinicial studies, directly relevant to clinical practice (which might interest the public as well as health professionals); preliminary studies in basic science, where scientists were addressing their peers; preliminary observations in clinical medicine; and more rigorous editorials, preferably based on meta-analyses founded on strict criteria. All this, Warren pointed out, would be merely to add a third tier to Sir Theodore Fox's original concept of recorder and newspaper functions of journals.[7]

Another suggestion was to add supplements reporting basic science to general clinical journals. But neither Relman nor Angell could agree to any of this. For most articles, they stated, information could not be classified in such a way—and they argued that a general medical journal should fight against the current fragmentation and superspecialisation of medicine; without a general viewpoint doctors would become plumbers rather than professionals. And, as Relman reminded us, there was a good claim for anecdotal case reports—important conditions such as primary aldosteronism had been first described in this format—and Richard Smith emphasised the danger of applying rigid ivory tower guidelines to research done under different circumstances, such as primary care. Journals, particularly general ones, serve a useful function by publishing a great variety of articles at different levels of interest and quality.

Inevitably the question of new formats surfaced, ranging from new types of printed texts such as *ACP Journal Club* (collected structured abstracts) and *Journalwatch* (summaries of articles with expert commentaries) through full texts on line or on CD-ROMs, to meta-analyses continuously updated in an electronic system. Self-evidently there are problems with all of these. The new printed formats had not yet been evaluated at the time of the seminar, but Franklin summarised some of the pros and cons of the new technology. On the one hand, three quarters of students in the developed world were computer literate, complex research such as the current human genome project was unthinkable without the use of computers, and many authors were no longer writing traditional articles—giving instead the background to the study and the data with only a very brief interpretation.

On the other hand, there were several difficulties with the new technology. The first was technical: the large variety of hardware and software serving the new developments needed standardising, and there were still difficulties in formatting tables and graphs if these were offered on line. Peer review of articles in an electronic format was difficult, given that complex items such as DNA sequences had to be recorded before they could be assessed; an algorithm for the accuracy of such sequences was, however, being developed. Electronic journals would be expensive, and, apart from workers in the pharmaceutical industry, would readers be prepared to pay up to $50 for a single article, as against $300 for an annual subscription to a journal? Expense also worked against the Third World, where in any case developments such as bibliographical databases on CD-ROMs were useless unless backed up with a fax machine that would deliver the full text. And surveys showed that given the choice readers still opted for the written text from the library rather than calling up the electronic version, and several discussants mentioned the loss if there was to be no more browsing through journals. Finally, how could scientific kudos be achieved with the new type of publication, where authors would achieve less visibility?

A major theme running through the seminar was whether it was placing excess emphasis on the responsibility of journals in improving information transfer. After all, Relman argued, what we know about how clinical practice changes suggests that the process is very complex: drug advertising and marketing, in particular, have powerful effects on what doctors do—much more than the results of the latest randomised controlled double blind trial. The problem, he argued, is not with journals: it is the habit of mind of doctors inadequately trained in rational analysis and the application of information.

Relman's arguments and indeed much of the discussion at the seminar underlined what every journal editor knows: our practices are largely empirical and unsupported by the results of rigorous research. We could start by attempting some definitions. What is our goal? What is the outcome measure? What is a 'good' journal—and good for whom, given that the needs of the health economist must differ from those of the medical student? So, though it is a common gibe that most articles finish with the cliché 'more research is needed,' that must also be the conclusion of the Leeds Castle seminar. Fortunately many of the editors present had research projects in train and further original work should be presented at the second world conference on peer review in 1993. Despite some scepticism, the results of such research must surely be helpful. For if, in John Ziman's words, the object of science truly is publication, then editors and the scientific community need a better basis for much of what they are currently doing.

1 de Solla Price D. The development and structure of the biomedical literature. In: Warren KS, ed: *Coping with the biomedical literature*. New York: Praeger, 1981;3–16.
2 Hamilton DP. Research papers: Who's uncited now? *Science* 1991;**251**:25
3 Gore SM, Jones IG, Rytter EC. Misuse of statistical methods: critical assessment of articles in BMJ from January to March 1976. *Br Med J* 1977;i:85–7.
4 Gardner MJ, Bond J. An exploratory study of statistical assessment of papers published in the British Medical Journal. *JAMA* 1990;**263**:1355–7.
5 Williamson JW, Goldschmidt PG, Colton T. The quality of medical literature: an analysis of validation assessments. In: Bailar JC, Mosteller F. *Medical use of statistics*. Waltham, Massachusetts: NEJM Books, 1986.
6 Williamson JW, German PS, Weiss R, Skinner EA, Bowes F. Health science information management and continuing education of physicians. A survey of US primary care practitioners and their opinion leaders. *Ann Intern Med* 1989;**110**: 151–60.
7 Fox TF. *Crisis in communication: the functions and future of medical journals*. London: Athlone Press, 1965.

PART 1
THE VOCATION/THE PROFESSION

A clinical scientist among the editors

CHRISTOPHER C BOOTH

The first issue of *Chiasma*, the official publication of the St Andrews University Medical Society, was published in the spring of 1949. The editorial was remarkable in its expression of the brimming over confidence of youth.[1] The journal was to be 'a reflection of what was happening in the minds of its readers', as they were also its contributors. It was to be 'a record of the past, an observer of the present, a prophet of the future, and an inevitable excursionist into the realms of fantasy'. It was to bring the ideas of the individual before the minds of the many. The functions of an editor were also considered in that brash editorial. The editorial chair, it was pointed out, should 'not be too comfortable, lest its occupant became too lethargic to carry out his editorship with success; nor must it indeed be too hard, for its hardness may penetrate the consciousness of the editor, who may become merciless in censorship or rejection. It would be useful if it were one of those chairs that swivel around, for it could then be turned to whatever direction it need be and could both formulate trends and follow them'. Despite the retreat from idealism which supposedly comes with advancing years, I have to confess that the concepts I then expressed of the function of a medical journal, and of the purposes of its editor, have not changed radically more than 40 years later.

It has, however, to be admitted that student medical journalism was no real apprenticeship for the highly competitive world of medical science that I entered five years later when I started clinical research at the Postgraduate Medical School at Hammersmith. We began with the preparation of case reports or of minor pieces of physiological investigation. Whatever was written was subjected to stringent review by our superiors and there might be pungent comments by the head of the department. Finally, after countless

11

and laborious redraftings and retypings, a typescript was despatched to a journal, in those days usually either the *British Medical Journal*, the *Lancet*, or (for more scientific endeavours) *Clinical Science*. It was then that you encountered for the first time the rejection letter, often immaculately phrased and in the case of the *Lancet* written with, as Stephen Lock has put it, 'an ethos of courtesy and emollience' that is unique to that remarkable journal.[2] I believe that I am unique in having received from the editor of the *Lancet* both a rejection and an acceptance in the same envelope. The first letter read:

This article is beautifully written, and I am loth to let it go. The tears that I pour over it as it leaves the office are not crocodile's. Any issue of *The Lancet* would be much improved by the inclusion of this paper; my one and only reason for parting with it is that we simply cannot cope with all that we should like to. Pray forgive me.

Pinned to that letter was another of the following day's date. To my delight it was a recantation:

I had dictated and signed a letter refusing your treatise . . . After a storm-tossed night I find that it is more than I can do to dispatch the intended letter. In a word, I look forward to publishing the paper—which only shows that even editors have bursts of conscience—or good sense.

By then I had become a professor, but at the outset of your career it would be rare indeed to be treated with such generous indulgence. At length, however, a paper would be accepted and there would follow that moment of high excitement when proofs arrived, the carefully crafted text set out in type, with a bewildering array of correction symbols listed on an accompanying sheet. I do not think that I have ever learnt to correct proofs according to the rules, but have always simply made sufficient scribbles to make clear where an error was detected—by methods that often must have been as bewildering to the printer as his instructions were to me. Proofs rapidly returned, you awaited with mounting excitement the actual publication. And then, so often, disappointment. You would walk into lunch with head held high to find that none of your colleagues had even noticed that from today you were an author.

Those far off days of the 1950s in Britain were to be associated with the founding of a series of important specialist journals to which the aspiring clinical scientist would increasingly contribute. I was privileged to appear in the early volumes of three of them. One of the most important was the *British Journal of Haematology*, which first came out in 1955. It was a journal that enjoyed immediate success, largely due to the exacting standards of its first editor. R G Macfarlane, the pioneer of studies of disorders of the clotting mechanism, modestly considered that one of his greatest contributions to haematology had been to persuade Sir John Dacie to become that first editor.[3] A clinical scientist of great distinction, later to be elected to the Fellowship of the Royal Society, Dacie not only insisted on the highest scientific standards but also imbued the journal with his own meticulous and perfectionist approach to correct presentation and accuracy in proof reading. As Per Saugman, his publisher at Blackwells, has written, he 'simply could not accept anything less than perfection.' He went on: 'A morning with him left one totally exhausted.' I remember a distinguished American visitor, finding him on one occasion in his room at Hammersmith painstakingly correcting commas and full stops, who remarked how extraordinary it was that such a mind should occupy itself with such minutiae. Yet it was that total dedication to such matters that gave the *British Journal of Haematology* so successful a start. There was no shortage of material to publish. Dacie, then head of the department in which I was carrying out research with D L Mollin, was also scrupulous in giving no unfair advantage to his own staff in terms of priority of publication. I recall in particular one paper which was nearly nine months in the pipeline,[4] a situation that we found profoundly disturbing for it very nearly resulted in our being overtaken by our competitors in a very competitive world.

The second journal which was to have an important influence on my developing career was *Gut*, of which I was later to become editor myself. Founded in 1960 by the British Society of Gastroenterology in association with the *BMJ*, *Gut*'s leading light was Sir Francis Avery Jones, who guided the journal through its early years. Sir Francis was the most eminent clinical gastroenterologist of his generation. It was a period when gastroenterology was evolving from being a mainly clinical specialty into a scientific discipline. Sir Francis, however, ensured that *Gut* would remain a predominantly clinical journal. His qualities were entirely different from those of Sir John Dacie. I can even recall an *x* ray that was published upside down. But he was an outstanding editor who was highly successful in encouraging the clinical community to subscribe to the journal, both at home and overseas. *Gut* very soon became a leading international journal, although L J Witts never considered it to have

13

achieved the scientific distinction of the *British Journal of Haematology*. Avery, as he is affectionately known, was once asked how he accounted for the success of *Gut*. 'If I ever see the word rat or dog in the title of a paper', he replied, 'I cross it out'.

As I was at the same time cultivating an interest in the history of medicine, the third new journal to which I was to contribute was *Medical History*, the first issues of which were published in 1957. It had an entirely different style from that of the scientific journals to which I and my then colleagues would contribute but, like both the *British Journal of Haematology* and *Gut*, its development owed everything to its early editors, one of whom was the distinguishd director of the Wellcome Institute of the History of Medicine, Dr Noel Poynter. I recall with pleasure the encouragement he gave to an amateur in a discipline in which Poynter himself was so towering a figure.

As time went on, I graduated from the position of author to that of reviewer. The first paper to arrive on your desk with a polite letter from an editor inviting an opinion is a great boost to the ego. There is also a distinct feeling that at last, after so many occasions which you have had to swallow hard and accept the views of some anonymous and unfriendly critic, you now have an opportunity to say your own piece. Frequently the paper would be from a competitor, and any unworthy temptation to be hypercritical and denigratory would have to be suppressed in favour of an attitude of creative criticism and encouragement. What the reviewer must consider is best summed up as follows:[5] Is it new? Is it true? And if it is, is it sufficiently important to warrant publication? Is it then appropriate for the journal to which it has been submitted? Finally, is it well enough written, a particular problem when the paper has been submitted by individuals whose native tongue is not English. Reviewing is a literary form that is never easy. Too often there is the temptation to rewrite according to your own style. Even more difficult, there is the tendency, encouraged by certain journals, to suggest further experiments which may or may not be relevant. The greatest difficulty, however, arises when the paper for consideration describes experiments similar to those that you are carrying out but the results of which you have not yet published. As in all human affairs, the behaviour of reviewers on such occasions is variable and not all follow the honourable course of returning the manuscript with a note declaring a conflict of interest. Journals and their editors are equally variable in their response to reviewers. It is, however, always gratifying to know the reaction to your opinion.

Many other literary duties fall to the lot of clinical scientists as they become increasingly established in their careers. They may be called on to write leading articles, report on meetings at home and abroad, write reviews of books or, increasingly in the modern era, comment on the issues of the day that impinge on the world of academe which they inhabit. The leading article is perhaps the most difficult of these tasks, demanding as it does a wide ranging review of the relevant literature, though that is so much easier today with modern library technology. Nevertheless, for many it is also considered the most rewarding for it gives an excellent opportunity to put their own work in perspective, untramelled by the views of people that they consider to be their detractors. Again there are temptations to be resisted. To ignore, impugn, or irresponsibly refute the work of competitors invites instant retribution in any journal that boasts a correspondence column.

Book reviewing is undoubtedly the most agreeable of these literary activities. It ensures that you actually read the book in question and, as you have probably been chosen as a reviewer because of your own particular interest in the subject matter, that does not usually prove difficult. I except from that generalisation the reviewing of massive textbooks, as when the editor of the *BMJ* was kind enough to permit me merely to skim the two volumes of the second edition of the *Oxford Textbook of Medicine*. The added bonus of book reviewing is that you are usually permitted to keep the book and thus avoid the expense of having to buy it. Frequently the authors of books you review write to you about what you have said. If the review was favourable, such correspondence may provide an uplift for the human spirit. With some diffidence I here give Sir Peter Medawar's response to what I said of his *Advice to a Young Scientist*,[6] but it was so characteristic of that noble and generous spirit that I am encouraged to record it. 'What an absolutely *marvellous* review', he wrote, 'I am so happy and grateful. It goes into the drawer marked "tonic"—to be opened when hypotheses are falsified or experiments go wrong.' Not all are so enthusiastic. I recall an American writer, a distinct zealot for his subject, who took me to task for criticising his habit of littering his typescript with quotations, some from holy writ, that were framed in black lines like pictures, a literary equivalent of those texts that adorned the walls of Victorian homes.

It is a wise rule never to write a review that is totally destructive. After all, the writing of any book is a literary achievement that all other practitioners of the art should regard with respect. Critics should also remember the advice of John Dryden. 'How easy it is to call rogue and villain', he wrote, 'and that wittily, but how hard to make a man appear a fool, a blockhead or a knave without using any of those opprobrious terms. There is still a vast difference betwixt the slovenly butchering of a man and the fineness of a stroke that separates the head from the body and leaves it standing in its place.'[7] I have only once written an uncompromisingly critical review. The work was historical and apart from its other shortcomings was seriously flawed by a series of appalling schoolboy howlers. I remember that my original draft began with two hackneyed quotations from Alexander Pope's *Essay on Criticism*—'Fools rush in where angels fear to tread' and 'A little learning is a dangerous thing'. Neither of these appeared in the final version but I was permitted the third of Pope's remembered epigrams from that same Essay—'To err is human, to forgive divine'. I have treasured ever since the page and a half of close typed vituperation that I received from the author.

The major problem facing the clinical investigator who undertakes these activities, which are additional to his major task of publishing the results of his own experimental work, is that they are always accompanied by deadlines. Deadlines are the lifeblood of journalists but to the investigator they hang like swords of Damocles over his spirit until the script is mercifully despatched. A gentle threat, however, is a splendid spur to literary activity.

There comes to many sooner or later a request to join the editorial board of a particular journal. The task varies from total involvement in the editorial process to mere attendance at an annual meeting and perhaps an increase in the amount of refereeing to be undertaken. For the privileged few, there is later the invitation to take over the editorship, a responsibility that is both an honour bestowed by their colleagues and a delight. For myself, the years that I spent as editor of *Gut*, from 1975 to 1981, were stimulating and rewarding, even though there were, it must be admitted, moments that might be regarded as acrimonious.

Gastroenterology during that period had become increasingly accepted as an academic discipline in this country. Refereeing when I took over was limited to a single opinion, together with that of the editor. I always used two referees. If they agreed about either acceptance or rejection their opinions usually, but by no means always, held sway. There were certain subjects on which I always exercised caution, such as when someone had shown that a drug might have a favourable effect on some obscure form of experimental liver damage in the rat. Such papers frequently had a commercial stigma attached to them. If the referees disagreed I often asked a member of the editorial board to adjudicate.

It was important then, as now, to ensure that the board maintained a balance between basic scientists and clinicians, and at that time we did not hesitate to publish papers about experimental work in animals. There was also a pressing need for expertise in statistics and I was fortunate in being able to recruit to the board David Hill, then secretary of the Royal Statistical Society and the son of Sir Austin Bradford Hill. I recall on one occasion that he was so concerned about the material with which he was confronted that he asked, and was granted, permission to recalculate the raw data of the individuals who had submitted a paper. We were then in a strong position to reject.

The greatest problem with reviewing was obtaining opinions within a reasonable time. In my time as editor we kept a blacklist of reviewers that we considered unreliable. Quite apart from those who actually lose manuscripts, there are reviewers who seem to tuck papers away in their brief-cases, hide them in their desks, scatter the pages on holiday beaches, or simply allow them to gather moss. They usually respond to the stimulus of a pained letter of encouragement. There was one, I recollect, who did not. After months of letters, recorded deliveries, telegrams, and telephone calls, I made a final effort. On the telephone I got the usual response that he was busy, on this occasion witnessing a procedure in the operating theatre. I asked his secretary if she would be kind enough to tell him that it was BBC television on the line. He came at once.

There is also the problem of whether there are individuals like Sir William Osler who take delight in hoaxes. (Osler's famous fabrication of the character of Egerton Y Davis, author of 'Professional notes among the Indian tribes about G Slave Lake, NWT', was a hoax played on the editors of the *Canada Medical and Surgical Journal*.)[8] When *Gut* was sent a paper entitled 'Scanning electron microscopy of the surface of the normal human stool', I have to confess—and it may have been unworthy—that I had my doubts. The aspiring contributor to whom I expressed those doubts, a fibre buff, responded by sending me a bag of bran.

Then there is the question of fraud. I can only confess that during my time as an editor I had no inkling that anything we published might have been based upon fraudulant data. As a recent article in the *Chicago Tribune* on the AIDS quest has shown,[9] however, possible or alleged fraud may only be revealed by a quality of

17

investigative journalism that is not available to the editor of a medical journal. Furthermore, whereas the United States has a Freedom of Information Act which permits the examination of laboratory notebooks, no such freedom is available in Britain. Unlike clinical records, the laboratory notebooks of scientists tend to be regarded as privileged documents in this country, which has always delighted in secrecy. Nevertheless, there must be many editors other than myself, advised by their referees, who have instinctively reacted against suspect material and therefore declined an offering.

There is no doubt about the success of the vast majority of the medical journals that have been founded during the past 40 years. They have been a reflection of developments during these past decades which have witnessed a centrifugal fragmentation of medicine into more and more parts. New scientific discoveries and new techniques have led to the development of more and more subspecialties in medicine. Each group practicing in these specialties has sought its own identity, often by establishing its own specialist society or in Britain its own Royal College. These groups then organise their own training programme so that they may control entry into their specialty. And inevitably they contribute to the increase in numbers of medical journals by founding their own subspecialty journal, the publication of which is also controlled by the same peer group. Most new journals in recent years have therefore been devoted to the organ orientation of the specialist group that founded them so that, although there is not yet to my knowledge a journal devoted to the great toe, we now have journals that cover all the organ systems of the body. Now, however, these journals are beginning to find themselves in something of a quandary. Advances in medicine axiomatically reflect advances in science and technology, and medical journals must therefore reflect the need for practitioners and scientists to work together in creative harmony. Such a situation was relatively easy to encourage when science, like medicine, was fragmenting. Editorial boards, for example, might include clinicians and basic scientists in the relevant discipline. Relatively suddenly all this is changing. Science, unlike medicine, is no longer fragmenting but converging. The Nobel laureate Arthur Kornberg perceived this paradox when he pointed out that the most profound development in medical science in recent years has been 'the confluence of many discrete and previously unrelated science subjects into a single unified discipline. Anatomy, physiology, biochemistry, microbiology, immunology, and genetics have now been merged and are being expressed in a common language. . . . by reducing structures and systems into molecular forms, all aspects of body form and function blend into a logical framework'.

For this reason many of the specialty groups, and the journals they control, have become heavily oriented towards technology and have tended to lose touch with modern science. Major clinical discoveries are being made not by the specialty group itself but by scientists working in other disciplines who publish not in specialty journals but in the major general journals of medicine and science. Though there is clearly a pressing need for maintaining links between science and the general medical journals, it is even more necessary for the specialist journals to rethink their scientific relations if they are to keep their readership accurately informed. If not, they will be relegated to the type of technical journal that is entirely inappropriate to serving the purposes of a learned profession.

For the future, however, if journals are to continue to engage the interest of their readers people who practise either science or medicine, or both, must be able to express themselves felicitously in print. I am not one who thinks that the publishing of books or journals will be replaced by modern electronic technology. Whatever happens, people will still have to face an empty page or a blank visual display unit when they seek to set out those individual views that they wish to convey to the many. Medawar, a superlative practitioner of the literary art, has written that most scientists 'write as if they hate writing and wanted above all else to have done with it'.[10] There have been medical grandees whose patrician prose evokes admiration but it has to be admitted that today they are a *rara avis*. The art of writing can, however, both be learnt and be improved by practice. I recall that in that editorial in *Chiasma* of so long ago, seeking to encourage literary activity among medical students at the University of St Andrews, I quoted the exhortation of Sir Arthur Quiller-Couch to his students in Cambridge: 'Literature being an Art', he had told them, 'part of our business is to practise it'. For the clinical scientist writing is often as great a chore as it is for any other scientist, but the relationship between an academic such as me and the editor of a medical journal is in fact creative. I regard that relationship as somewhat similar to that between an undergraduate and his tutor. The tutor, who is the editor, sets me essays to write, reserving to himself the right to make whatever judgement he will. There are those who bridle at any criticism of their solicited efforts. For myself, however, I—and I was going to say grudgingly, but I think that reluctantly will do—

19

express my gratitude to the many editors of medical journals who have tormented me with requests for copy, distorted my manuscripts, corrected my grammar, criticised my syntax, disturbed my sleep with concern about deadlines, and in other ways persuaded me to follow Sir Arthur Quiller-Couch's advice by rousing me from my innate literary lethargy. In particular, I express my gratitude to my taskmaster of today, Dr Stephen Lock, editor of the journal whose 150th anniversary we are now celebrating.

1 Booth CC. *Chiasma. The official publication of the St Andrews University Medical Society* [Editorial]. 1949;**1**:3–4.
2 Lock SP. Declination: the art of courteous editorial rejection. In: *Swerving neither to the right nor the left*. London: The Keynes Press, 1988:29–32.
3 Saugman P. *From the first fifty years. An informal history of Blackwell Scientific Publications*. Oxford: Blackwell, 1989:23.
4 Booth CC, Chanarin I, Anderson BB, Mollin DL. The site of absorption and tissue distribution of orally administered 56Co-labelled vitamin B12 in the rat. *Br J Haematol* 1957;**3**:253–61.
5 Lock SP. *A difficult balance: editorial peer review in medicine*. London: The Nuffield Provincial Hospitals Trust, 1985:7–8. Reprinted London: BMJ, 1991.
6 Booth CC. Uplift for the spirit. *Br Med J* 1980;**280**:1081–2.
7 Cook RI. *Sir Samuel Garth*. Boston: Twayne, 1980:73.
8 Cushing H. *The life of Sir William Osler*. Oxford: Clarendon Press, 1925:**1**:181.
9 Special report. The great AIDS quest. *Chicago Tribune*, November 19, 1989.
10 Medawar PB. *Advice to a young scientist*. New York: Harper and Row, 1979:63.

As things really were?

STEPHEN LOCK

At times I feel that all editors are caught up in a ritual dance whose pace is continually accelerating, similar to that in the final scene of Ingmar Bergman's film *The Seventh Seal*, where in a long line the major characters join hands together with Death. More than ever scientific journals are an integral part of scientific research, a conclusion that carries two major implications. Firstly, journals now achieve greater visibility and cachet than they did. Secondly, journals have had thrust upon them new responsibilities and duties not only to the scientific community but also to society, which ultimately pays for them and is concerned in their standards.

We thought that one way to commemorate the 150th anniversary of the *British Medical Journal* would be to look at current and future problems, the achievement of scientific journals and their likely future agenda. Given that the editors of four of the world's principal general medical journals had just retired or were about to do so, there was a golden opportunity to get them and their successors together with other invited experts to discuss these issues.

Here I consider developments in journals in four phases. The first is the period to the end of the second world war. The second, from 1945 to 1979, saw the flowering of modern clinical science and almost universal peer review for scientific journals.[1] The third, 1980 to 1990, is set against a backdrop of high inflation rates and a slowing down in scientific research funding. During this time the computer came into its own in helping to develop a new discipline—citation analysis[2]—which is still being argued about today, and in being applied to sophisticated retrieval and document delivery systems. But much more important was the discovery of a new threat—misconduct in scientific research—a watershed in the evolution of journals, given that it thrust them under a spotlight. This forced editors to appraise concepts such as duplicate and 'excessive' publication, authorship, and conflicts of interest and how to put the

21

record straight in proved fraud. It also meant a close examination of peer review and other editorial practices, to see whether misconduct could have been detected earlier, and it is why I separate these ten years off as a distinct period.

The final phase I shall consider briefly is the future. My thesis is that in the 300 years of their existence journals have done too little to examine their own practices. If, as many think, research is incomplete without publication—exemplified by Ziman's 'The object of science is publication'[3] or Faraday's 'Work, finish, publish'[4]—then we could generalise Ingelfinger's statement about peer review to the study of scientific editing: the irony, as he pointed out, that 'material often obtained in the most rigorous kind of biomedical experimentation is rated as publishable or not by a system that has rarely been subjected to any analysis, let alone one that is rigorous'.[5]

Before 1945

Scientific journals started in 1665 with the publication of two that are still extant: the *Journal de Scavans*, produced by the French Academy, and the *Philosophical Transactions of the Royal Society*. The standards of these and other early journals was variable, but from the beginning several relied on peer review of original articles.[6] Moreover, by the mid-nineteenth century both the content of the journal and the structure of the article had come to resemble their present day counterparts. Thus, 125 years ago, the *BMJ* contained a mixture of information (original articles), instruction (editorials), comment (letters to the editor), and miscellanea (with an impressive coverage of news events all over the world).[7] The original articles do not consistently have the IMRAD structure (Introduction, Methods, Results, and Discussion)—in particular, the summary or abstract developed late, appearing sporadically in the early 1920s and regularly in the '40s[8]—but the narrative is logical and has an accompanying apparatus of illustrations and tables, as well as of references, which began to be collected together at the end of articles from 1877.

This was the pattern of most general journals until the end of the second world war. Perhaps their three striking features today are the preponderance of printed orations and lectures by the medical good and the great—in effect review articles, though they usually include more personal experience than today's equivalents—the anecdotal nature of most of the clinical reports, and the anonymity of many features that would now be signed, such as book reviews, editorials, and even many letters to the editor.

Another major development in the century before 1945 was the publication of specialist journals. A few of these began as early as the 1820s and '30s and by the second part of the nineteenth century several of today's major journals had been started (including the *American Journal of Obstetrics*, *Brain*, *Annals of Surgery*, and *Journal of Pathology*).[9] All this led to the realisation that the number of journals was increasing both regularly and rapidly and some scientists became concerned at the 'information explosion'. In 1939 the British physicist J D Bernal suggested that drastic action should be taken to restrict this growth, proposing that journals should be classified into archival or recorder publication and newspaper or current awareness journals.[10] The former could even be replaced, Bernal went on, by a system of distributing abstracts of articles sent to a central source, with interested readers obtaining copies of the full paper on request.

Nevertheless, by today's standards the total number of biomedical journals was not uncomfortably high (around 4000 in 1950). Partly this was because many journals ceased publication, particularly in the nineteenth century; at the end of this one count showed that, of the 1147 ever begun, only 250 were still being published (and no fewer than 339 of the 386 journals published in Germany and Austria had ceased to appear).[9] But mostly it was because biomedical research had yet to achieve today's dominant position with its large investment in workers and materials and output of increasingly specialised findings, which needed publication. Publication also sometimes came to have a different role, with articles duplicated or fragmented to swell a curriculum vitae or an annual departmental report. These were to be prominent features of the subsequent periods, and the exponential growth and differentiation of journals became a subject for research, with an ingenious concept to explain why these had come about.[11]

1945–79

War is renowned for provoking enormous advances in all forms of technology and in both world wars medicine benefited hugely. Nevertheless, it is a mistake to look for a sharp dividing line: rather, as the journals show, medicine evolved steadily from the anecdotal to the more rigorous—from the concept of the Bull Borst regimen for treating crush injuries from air raids, for example, to the early

23

coil haemodialysers and then today's complex dialysis machines, or from the anecdotal reports in the 1940s about the efficacy of the new but crude penicillin preparations in battle injuries to the postwar trials of the use of the purified product in civilian illnesses (revolutionising the outlook, say, in subacute bacterial endocarditis).

After the war many of the antibiotics and other new products, such as cortisone or pertussis vaccine, were in short supply or their efficacy was undetermined—hence proper evaluation was needed. It was now that the statisticians came into their own (although discussion of probability had appeared in two general medical journals as early as 1934 and 1936, with a series of articles on statistics in medicine in 1937.[12-14] Journals came to print numerous reports of randomised double blind controlled trials, few articles containing data seemed to be without p values in parentheses, while a series of exciting epidemiological reports disclosed unknown links—between cigarette smoking and lung cancer, chronic bronchitis, and coronary artery disease, for example, or between x irradiation and acute leukaemia. And there were the exciting discoveries of new entities, such as aldosterone and other hormones, let alone the emergence of disciplines such as immunology which paved the way to clinical applications such as organ transplantation.

The intensity of the activity in clinical science was mirrored in the journals. The format of original articles now assumed its modern guise;[8] the IMRAD formula was universal as was a summary at the end of the article (in the 1960s to change its position to the beginning and its name to abstract); tables and illustrations were more frequent and prepared by professionals; and there was some internal consistency to the references—often, but not always, in what the British had christened the 'Harvard' system, giving the authors' names and publication dates in the text and alphabetically at the end of the article.[15]

Given the pace and variety of these new concepts, editors came to have new responsibilities. Largely gone was any lackadaisical approach typified by Virchow, who had claimed that anybody was free to make a fool of himself in his journal.[16] Work now needed to be certified as reasonable and credible; hence editors relied increasingly on peer review of articles by experts (although this did not become universal until the late 1950s).[6] Articles had to be made as clear as possible for the non-expert; hence these were more heavily subedited to make the language and the message easier to assimilate—particularly important now that English had replaced German as the international language of science and an increasing number of non-anglophone workers were having to write and read articles in English.

New findings also had to be explained and put into perspective for the non-specialist reader, an aim most readily achieved through commissioning editorial and review articles. Finally, if some tentative findings were supported by other research groups and had implications for public policy then the editor needed to consider running a campaign. This had been a feature of medical journals in Victorian times—Wakley of the *Lancet* pressing for medical reform, for example, or Hart of the *BMJ* for laws against infanticide—but had largely disappeared by the 1940s. Now, with the demonstration, say, that expensive specialised care and facilities could save the lives of premature babies, or that cigarette smoking was killing thousands of citizens prematurely every year, editors again recognised their wider duty to society and need to persuade its leaders of the case for action.

All these changes affected editorial philosophies.[17] Journals became more user friendly. Thus, whereas traditionally the editor's decision about publication of an article had been final, usually with no reasons for rejection given, the authors could now challenge the verdict, particularly if the referees' comments were sent, as they increasingly were. Again, journals began to abandon anonymity, at first for book reviews, then for news items, and finally for editorials. Given that in many countries the state was now providing health care, medicine increasingly came to have an important political role (with a small 'p') and comments in journals a heightened visibility; many readers felt that to know who was putting something forward might be almost as important as what he was saying—at least any possible conflict of interest might become apparent.

The one aspect where anonymity was retained was peer review, editors arguing that this ensured franker opinions.[18] Yet even here some journals came to allow referees to sign their reports if they wished (an option taken up by about 15% of them).[19]

Lastly editors came to audit their activities and to apply the result to raising the standards of journals, sometimes by requiring clinical scientists to improve their own standards. Thus immediately after the war there were disquieting revelations about medical research in the Nazi concentration camps resulting in the production of the Nuremberg code. In the mid-1950s concern grew about clinical research on human subjects without informed consent. In Britain this culminated in *Human Guinea Pigs*, a well documented book;[20] reports by the Royal College of Physicians, the Medical Research

Council, and the Ministry of Health leading to setting up research ethics committees;[21] and an international code of practice. The last—the World Medical Association's Declaration of Helsinki— was drawn up by the editors of two general medical journals (Hugh Clegg of the *BMJ* and Tapani Kosonen of the *Finnish Medical Journal*) and was a further guide to researchers.[22] It also enabled editors to monitor the ethical standards of work submitted for publication, as well as to comment on that already published. A similar code about studies on animals was produced a few years later.

A further type of audit was of what many readers had come to take on trust—the statistical aspects of a published study. In 1966, two decades after the 'statistical revolution', two American statisticians chose 10 of the most frequently read American medical journals and asked experienced biostatisticians to read 25 articles in each:[23] were the conclusions valid for the design of the experiment, what about the type of analysis, and were the statistical tests applicable? The group found widespread faults, with no fewer than 12 types of error, though most of the conclusions still stood. Clearly expert help was needed and slowly journals on both sides of the Atlantic started to introduce a separate statistical check once an article had been provisionally approved for publication—particularly after similar surveys had shown statistical errors of commission or omission or both in other journals or widespread deficiencies in the reports of clinical trials, therapeutic trials, and drug side effects.[6]

Another theme surfaced again during the latter part of this period: the relation between an editor and the owners of the journal. At various annual meetings of the BMA in the nineteenth and early twentieth century editors of the *BMJ* such as Hart and Dawson Williams had survived threats of censure, or even calls for their dimissal—and the same was true of editors elsewhere, though some were dismissed, such as James Warbase, of the *New York State Journal of Medicine* who in 1908 fell out with his board over advertising policy.[24] In the 1950s there was talk of continual difficulties between Morris Fishbein, editor of *JAMA*, and the AMA (and in 30 years in another country there were no fewer than nine different full time editors of a national medical journal). Nevertheless, only one of the modern challenges is well documented. In 1958 Hugh Clegg, then editor of the *BMJ*, angered the BMA establishment by attacking the Royal College of Physicians. It was claimed, untruly, that he had contravened BMA policy. His editorial was censured by the BMA Council, which also attempted to restrict his activities, but the customary editorial freedom was reconfirmed and restored by the next Annual Representative Meeting, the policy making body of the BMA.[25] [26] It is worth quoting the BMA By-laws, which now state categorically, 'A journal, under the title of the British Medical Journal, shall be published by or on behalf of the Association, and shall be conducted by a paid Editor, who shall be responsible for all that appears therein . . .'

Given all these developments and preoccupations, not surprisingly editors closed ranks, forming groups and organisations. To be sure, editors of major journals had always had colleagues to talk to, but most journals were still edited on a shoestring by academics working part time in their university departments. They felt isolated and ignorant of the new developments; nor were such attitudes exclusive to medical editors, and hence the new organisations were broadly based.[17] The Council of Biology Editors (CBE) was formed in the USA in 1957, and its European counterpart, ELSE (Earth and Life Science Editing), 10 years later, subsequently being retitled EASE (European Association of Science Editors). Both developed style and other instruction manuals, and continue to publish regular bulletins and hold assemblies and courses, activities which are evidently popular, given the high current membership figures. Apart from a highly successful African editors' organisation, however, attempts to form similar bodies elsewhere (such as in Australia or South East Asia), have not produced lasting organisation, probably because of the lack of money or sufficient numbers of potential members or the difficulties in travelling large distances.

Despite these moves, at the end of this period several full time medical editors thought that an umbrella organisation was needed for medicine. This had particular problems and medical journals were in the majority in both CBE and EASE. The idea was brought to a head when a secretary publicly complained about the load imposed by the numerous reference styles, each specific for one medical journal.[27] Ten journals agreed to standardise reference styles for 18 journals and it was then proposed to extend the scope of this agreement. Four editors met during a conference at Atlantic City and one agreed to produce a draft of instructions to authors for debate; the final version could then be proposed for universal application.[28] Independently I had been discussing with two American editors the need for a small professional group to consider the specific needs of medicine. Several of us were present at a meeting of several Canadian major medical organisations at Vancouver in January 1979, and hence the International Committee of Medical

27

Journal Editors (the Vancouver group) was born. This produced a document of instructions for authors (jocularly known as the Declaration of Vancouver[29] [30]) and at its regular meetings since has gone on to consider a variety of issues.

The final topic to consider here is the growth of scientific journals. Here our guru is Derek de Solla Price, who in 1961 showed that there was no information 'explosion': the rate of expansion since the beginning of serious publication in 1665 had been a constant 5–7% a year.[11] Moreover, there was a constant ratio of the number of journals per scientist, which had not changed over the past 30 years—a suggestion confirmed more recently by other research.

de Solla Price's rule of thumb was that a scientist who publishes one article a year can take in the contents of more than one other paper a month but less than one article a day. Hence the formation of 'invisible colleges'—networks of a few hundred scientists publishing for each other. Disciplines tend to split every 10 years or so, and the new subdisciplines do not necessarily correspond with the organisational and professional structures. The new subdisciplines need new journals, where authorship and readership are often identical, while the old journals of the original disciplines continue to be published for a wide readership, which is far larger than the authorship.[31] In this way the general and specialist journals come to form a hierarchy of general scientific/general medical/specialist/super-specialist/super-super-specialist/and so on—recently added to by the non-peer reviewed 'grey literature' of preprints, handouts, fax messages, and electronic mail.

Nevertheless, journals have also changed to meet the needs of their readership and their disciplines.[17] General journals have become more newsy, returning in editorial and feature articles to a concern about social issues, such as funding health care and prison medicine. Specialist journals in the first tier have become the general journal of their discipline, with editorials, review articles, and opinion pieces, instead of the unvaried diet of original papers only a few years ago. In this way somebody working in a subdiscipline, say, paediatric genetics, can keep in touch with developments in the general specialty or other paediatric subspecialties. And there have been experiments with electronic journals or the storage of reserve data in an electronic form.

de Solla Price's model is attractive for its consistency and neatness, yet I have always been worried about some of the details. In particular, where did he get his figures from, and just how many journals are published in various countries, especially in the Third

World? For example, on the basis of records in *Ulrich's International Periodical Directory* it has been claimed that de Solla Price's exponential growth in journal numbers is finally slowing down.[32]. Though this could be predicted in any 'biological' system, *Ulrich* does not include several journals with visibility. Thus one of my priorities would be a rigorous survey of true journal numbers all over the world—a difficult task given the number of journals with restricted local circulations and intermittent appearance. Despite these reservations, however, nobody has suggested a more plausible scheme for the growth of science and of the journals that serve it.

1980–90

In 1980 a percipient reader noted that an article in a Japanese journal written by Elias K Alsabti was identical to that written by K W Pettingale and D E H Tee published in the *Journal of Clinical Pathology*.[33] A literature search showed that Alsabti, a Jordanian doctor who had worked in the USA and the United Kingdom, had followed the same pattern in plagiarising at least 60 other articles. As an isolated occurrence this might have been used to illustrate the usual honesty of science—similar to other occasional aberrant work such as that of Cyril Burt on intelligent quotients or to the Piltdown man hoax. At the most it would have shown that peer review had been inadequate, though little harm had been done and the record could be put straight. But the Alsabti incident proved to be only the prologue to a series of revelations about numerous other research workers who had committed serious misconduct (a blanket term covering piracy, plagiarism, and fraud).

The scale of the individual misconduct was considerable: John Darsee, a Harvard research fellow in cardiology, had forged data in 44 original articles and over 100 abstracts,[34] Robert Slutsky, a University of California intern in radiology, in 12 articles.[35] In all from 1980 to 1990 over 20 cases of proved misconduct in medicine were documented in the USA, five in Australia, and five in Britain.[36] Yet this was almost certainly only the tip of a sizable iceberg: my anecdotal survey of 29 medical schools and other institutions in Britain disclosed 61 cases not in the public domain, while there were statements that the British regulatory authorities mistrusted 5% of any drug research done in general practice and an even higher proportion of that done elsewhere in Europe.[36]

One difficulty in studying misconduct has been in not knowing its prevalence; Koshland argued that only 1 in 100 000 pieces of scientific information were tainted,[37] whereas Broad and Wade suspected that there were very many concealed cases for every major overt instance.[38] Nevertheless, a survey of some of the major research bodies by one of the experts on misconduct, Pat Woolf, concluded that there was no evidence of an epidemic of fraud in the United States. Rather there was a persistent and growing concern about the conduct of science and its publication.[39] The former included 'sloppy' science—for example, inadequate record keeping and retention of data, supervision of trainees, and policies about controls (which might be historical or those already used in another piece of research without this being stated).

Above all, however, there was a prevailing faulty philosophy, with the emphasis on cutting corners and a hurried pace. And this also applied to publication practices. Whereas research suggested that an active researcher could produce two original articles and ten conference abstracts a year,[40] many well known (but honest) scientists had their names on several times this number while some fraudulent workers such as Slutsky were producing one original article every 10 days, with the only comment by his colleagues on their scale and diversity being approbation.[35] In his and other cases of misconduct this was accompanied by 'gift' authorship, putting colleagues' names on the papers, often but not always with their approval.

Another cause of the excessive number of articles per author and an ever increasing load on the retrieval services was duplicate publication—the identical article in a general journal and specialist journal, in a national and international journal, or in a journal and conference proceedings. Almost always the article was submitted without telling the editor of the secondary journal about the first article or giving a reference to it. A similar failure to inform was also a frequent feature of two other forms of unwelcome publication. In 'salami' publication the findings of a single study were split among several different journals; in 'meat extender' publication the author wrote a second article adding, say, a couple of additional patients to the original series, but with no new insights or conclusions.

Over this period there were two other disquieting practices. Firstly, the increasing tendency to release material that was already under consideration or in press in a medical journal to the public through the media, such as newspapers, radio, and television. Secondly, there were potential conflicts of interest. Authors might not disclose their financial involvement in a product, or the sources of financial or material support, or they might fail to cite work by rival workers; referees might give an opinion on an article while concealing similar links of their own.

At first the scientific community was slow in dealing with these challenges; its reaction to fraud, as Marcia Angell has stated, was characterised by confusion and a horror of going public.[41] Nevertheless, individual cases were investigated and the findings published, while the larger issues were tackled in a series of conferences and reports. Thus there are now two major documents from the USA on maintaining high ethical standards in research and investigating promptly and fairly any allegations of misconduct[42] [43] as well as a recent one from the United Kingdom.[44] The Vancouver group has discussed how journals could standardise published retractions,[45] and *Index Medicus* has developed a method of linking these with the original article on MEDLINE, also introducing the new MeSH term of RETRACTED PUBLICATION.[46]

Nevertheless, the official agencies have also been concerned in attempts at prevention. To the original suggestion about good laboratory practice have been added detailed proposals from the Institute of Medicine.[47] Editors have debated the criteria for authorship,[30] and some have started asking referees and authors to sign disclaimers of conflict of interest.[48] At least one university, Harvard, has suggested a limit on the number of articles job applicants may cite in their curricula vitae.[49] Not everybody will cooperate over these proposals. Some editors have refused to print retractions of fraudulent articles that have appeared in their journals, stating that they had no mechanism or that it was against editorial policy.[50] Some heads of academic departments have declined to use existing guidelines on authorship or even to consider drawing their own up (Huth EJ, personal communication, 1989).

Clearly, then, 1980–90 has been exceptionally active for scientific publication, but it has been marked by divergent attitudes of professionals and the public. Editors and scientists have long known that much in their journals will not survive; sorting out the material of permanent value from the rest was after all one of the original purposes of publication. They have recognised that peer review can often do no more than ensure that a paper is credible, prevent the publication of bad work, and improve the scholarship, language, and presentation of data. Nevertheless, these are important roles and the reason that editors frown on scientists releasing non-peer reviewed work to the media. Administrators and politicians, on the other hand, have taken an opposite stance. They have laid much emphasis on refereeing, using the phrase that an article has 'passed peer review' to imply some gold standard, or seal of approval. Nevertheless, it has become clear that peer review cannot be relied on to detect fraud; a few instances have been disclosed in this way but most have been detected by the shrewd observation of colleagues or by scientists who have tried to replicate the work.

The tensions between professional scientists (including editors) and managers have surfaced at the congressional hearings chaired by representative John Dingell—which have left the public with the impression that science and its practices are much too important to be left to the scientists. Thus the need for good editing practices is paramount, and these include audit and research into structure, process, and outcome. A start has been made with studies of some important aspects, particularly the first international conference on peer review held in Chicago in 1989,[51] but more needs to be done— and urgently if governments are not to step in and tell everybody concerned how to do their tasks. I will discuss some of these steps in the final section.

The future

In retrospect one of the amusing aspects of predictions is how wrong many of them prove to be. Thus we still have not achieved Bernal's suggestion about recorder and newspaper journals, subsequently to be enlarged on by Sir Theodore Fox.[52] Yet evolution takes much longer than anybody ever thinks and possibly we may now be nearer developing some sort of similar scheme. The structured abstract, I believe, is one of the most important concepts of the past decade.[53] By printing it and storing the remaining article electronically after the original script has undergone peer review the editor will do his readers two main services. Firstly, he will give most of them all that they want to read, without losing any of the academic rigour conferred by the full text (which may anyway become more rigorous in revision by giving more detail). Secondly, he will be able to find space for many more articles—both original (including replication and those with negative results) and review features, commenting on these and other original articles published elsewhere. If these reviews and editorials, moreover, are written with recently proposed guidelines in mind then their value should be even greater than the corresponding features today.[53]

This need to keep in touch with important developments is particularly important given that 'the literature' is now much wider:

compared with 30 years ago articles today now have references to twice the number of journals.[54] Almost certainly it explains the recent recrudescence of the abstracting journal, which featured in the mid 1940s. But the new abstracting journals are different: they are both critical and selective. The new approach (exemplifed by *Journalwatch* and *ACP Journal Club*) extends the McMaster philosophy that many demonstrably intellectually vapid articles are being published, even in the best journals, and that by a ruthless appraisal and eliminating the meretricious a reader can cut down the time he spends.[55] And surely editors will also want to go on narrowing the number of articles that are insufficiently valid to be published.

To be sure, some work can often be disproved only after publication, by analysis or failure of replication, yet much is still being published that more rigorous peer review would have shown is substandard. I believe that the wider use of checklists, together with an audit of the fate of published work, will help, but above all peer review has to be improved and the referee helped more. For example, we don't even have a definition of a peer reviewed journal yet, let alone a tracking study of manuscripts throughout a scientific community that might show just how things really are. One way of helping referees might be to use the electronic databases, doing a literature search for similar work before sending new articles to reviewers; another by more guidance on the advice editors want together with feedback on the article's fate. We also need to know whether, as has been stated, blind review truly results in better standards;[56] to use the inevitable cliché, further studies are urgently needed. All this is likely to be helped by continuing the international conferences on peer review; the next is due in September 1993.

Some will object that these changes will take the fun out of editing. I disagree: choosing original articles should be no more 'fun' than piloting a commercial aircraft—the pilot follows a series of sensible rules and checklists to achieve the best possible result for society. If he does not then society can take action, and I believe that eventually the same might be true for editors who accept an article that, for example, produces widespread public alarm but which has not been through an accepted editorial process—or, again, who refuse to set the record straight subsequently. The fun of editing will never disappear, but it comes from balancing and shaping a journal by injecting an individual approach. Given that this has been a feature for over 300 years, it is hardly likely to be

33

affected by a few more sensible guidelines, of which we need more rather than fewer.

1 Burnham JC. The evolution of editorial peer review. *JAMA* 1990;**263**:1323–9.
2 Garfield E. Citation analysis as a tool in journal evaluation. *Science* 1972;**178**:471–9.
3 Ziman J. *Public knowledge.* Cambridge: Cambridge University Press, 1968.
4 Faraday M. Cited by *JAMA* in 'flyer' leaflet for 1st international conference on peer review. Chicago: AMA, 1988.
5 Ingelfinger FJ. Peer review in biomedical publication. *Am J Med* 1974;**56**:686–92.
6 Lock S. *A difficult balance: editorial peer review in medicine.* London: Nuffield Provincial Hospitals Trust, 1985. Reprinted London: BMJ, 1991.
7 Bartrip P. *Mirror of medicine.* Oxford: Oxford University Press, 1990.
8 Smith J. Journalology—or what editors do. *BMJ* 1990;**301**:756.
9 Lock S. Medical journals. In: *Oxford companion to medicine.* Oxford: Oxford University Press, 1985.
10 Bernal JD. Provisional scheme for central distribution of scientific publications. Presented at Royal Society Scientific Information Conference, 1948. Reprinted in: Meadows AJ, ed. *The scientific journal.* London: Aslib, 1979.
11 de Solla Price D. *Science since Babylon.* New Haven: Yale University Press, 1961.
12 Mainland D. Chance and the blood count. *Can Med Assoc J* 1934;**30**:656–8.
13 Mainland D. Problems of chance in clinical trials. *Br Med J* 1936;ii:221–4.
14 Hill AB. *Principles of medical statistics*, 9th ed. London: Lancet, 1971.
15 Chernin E. The 'Harvard' system: a mystery dispelled. *Br Med J* 1988;**297**:1062–3.
16 Anonymous. Are referees a good thing? [editorial]. *Can Med Assoc J* 1974;**111**:897–8.
17 Lock S. 'Journalology': are the quotes needed? *CBE Views* 1989;**12**:57–9.
18 Relman AS. Are journals really quality filters? In: Goffman W, Bruer JT, Warren KS, eds. *Research on selective information systems.* New York: Rockefeller Foundation, 1980.
19 Relman AS. Reviewers and the peer review system. In: Warren KS, ed. *Coping with the biomedical literature.* New York: Praeger, 1981.
20 Pappworth MH. *Human guinea pigs: experimentation on man.* London: Routledge and Kegan Paul, 1967.
21 Ministry of Health. *Supervision of the ethics of clinical research.* London: HMSO, 1968. (HM(68)33).
22 Gilder S. World Medical Association meets in Helsinki. *Br Med J* 1964;ii:299–300.
23 Schor S, Karten I. Statistical evaluation of medical journal manuscripts. *JAMA* 1966;**195**:1123–8.
24 Warbase JP. Medical journalism. State journalism in particular: with especial reference to the New York state medical journal. *NY State J Med* 1908;**8**:599–601.
25 Anonymous. The gold-headed cane. *Br Med J* 1956;i:791–3.
26 Anonymous. BMA Annual Representative Meeting 1956: leading articles in the *Journal. Br Med J* 1956;ii (suppl):12–4.
27 Huth EJ. Uniform requirements for manuscripts. *Ann Intern Med* 1979;**90**:120.
28 Huth EJ. CBE will not be saved by grace alone, good works are needed. *CBE Views* 1987;**10**:55–7.
29 Anonymous. Declaration of Vancouver. *Br Med J* 1978;i:1302–3.
30 International Committee of Medical Journal Editors. Uniform requirements for manuscripts submitted to biomedical journals. *BMJ* 1991;**302**:338–41.
31 de Solla Price D. The development and structure of the biomedical literature. In:

Warren KS, ed. *Coping with the biomedical literature*. New York: Praeger, 1981; 3–16.

32 Pendlebury D. Science's go-go growth: has it started to slow? *New Scientist* 1986;7 August:14 and 16.

33 Anonymous. Must plagiarism thrive? *Br Med J* 1980;**281**:41–2.

34 Relman AS. Lessons from the Darsee affair. *N Engl J Med* 1983;**308**:1415–7.

35 Engler RL, Corell JW, Friedman PJ, Kitcher PS, Peters RM. Misrepresentation and responsibility in medical research. *N Engl J Med* 1987;**317**:1583–9.

36 Lock S. Misconduct in medical research: does it exist in Britain? *Br Med J* 1988;**297**:1531–5.

37 Koshland DE. Fraud in science. *Science* 1987;**235**:41.

38 Broad W, Wade N. *Betrayers of the truth*. New York: Simon and Shuster, 1982.

39 Woolf P. Fraud in science: how much, how serious? *Hastings Cent Rep* 1981;**11**:9–14.

40 Batshaw ML, Plotnick LP, Petty BG, Woolf PK, Milliks ED. Academic promotion at a medical school. *N Engl J Med* 1988;**318**:741–7.

41 Angell M. Fraud in science. *Science* 1982;**219**:1417–8.

42 Association of American Medical Colleges. *The maintenance of high ethical standards in the conduct of research. Report of ad hoc committee adopted by the executive council of the AAMC 24 June 1982*. Washington, DC: AAMC, 1982.

43 Association of American Universities. *Framework for institutional policies and procedures to deal with fraud in research*. Washington, DC: Association of American Universities, 1988.

44 Royal College of Physicians. *Fraud and misconduct in medical research*. London: Royal College of Physicians, 1991.

45 International Committee of Medical Journal Editors. Retraction of research findings. *Br Med J* 1988;**296**:400.

46 Anonymous. Retracted publication. *Cumulated Index Medicus*. Vol 30. Bethesda, Maryland: National Library of Medicine, 1989.

47 Institute of Medicine. *The responsible conduct of research in the health sciences*: Washington DC: National Academy Press, 1989.

48 Lundberg GD. Editorial freedom and integrity. *JAMA* 1988;**260**:2563.

49 Harvard Medical School. *Guidelines for investigators in scientific research*. Cambridge, Massachusetts: Harvard University, 1988.

50 Kohn A. *False prophets: fraud and error in science and medicine*. Oxford: Blackwell, 1986.

51 JAMA. Guarding the guardians: research on editorial peer review. *JAMA* 1990;**263**:1317–441.

52 Fox TF. *Crisis in communication: the functions and future of medical journals*. London: Athlone Press, 1965.

53 Ad Hoc Working Group for Critical Appraisal of the Medical Literature. A proposal for more informative abstracts of clinical articles. *Ann Intern Med* 1987;**106**:598–604.

54 Huth EJ. The information explosion. *Bull NY Acad Med* 1989;**65**:647–61.

55 Sackett DL. Evaluation: requirements for clinical application. In: Warren KS, ed. *Coping with the biomedical literature*. New York: Praeger, 1981.

56 McNutt RA, Evans TA, Fletcher RH, Fletcher SW. The effects of blinding on the quality of peer review. *JAMA* 1990;**263**:1355–7.

'Without truckling or pandering': the professionalisation of medical editing

PATRICIA K WOOLF

With all the trouble professions are in these days, it is not clear why any group would aspire to that status. Nevertheless, many different occupations have struggled to be, and to appear, more professional.[1] So it is important to understand that impulse and the distinction that being a 'profession' confers. To begin with, let us discuss several distinctions associated with professionalism that do not apply to medical editing. We all know that in sports, the distinction between 'professional' and 'amateur' formerly separated those who did it for money and those who did it for love. In modern times, it is clear that scientific editors are amateurs in the sense that most do it more for love than money.[2] Despite the precedents of medicine and the law, professionalism is not simply a matter of official certification or licensure. In America, egg graders are licensed in Indiana, horse shoers in Illinois, and well diggers in Maryland.[3] Proposals to certify editors are still in the planning stage and have focused on the more mechanical aspects of copy editing manuscripts. As most editors of medical journals are already professionals by virtue of being doctors, the important question is that of the consequences for medical editing if it is considered to be a separate or an emerging profession.

Celebratory occasions and anniversaries (such as this 150th anniversary of the *British Medical Journal*), however, provide opportunities for worthwhile reflection and assessment. In that spirit we shall discuss whether, and to what extent, the vocation or occupation of medical editing is a profession and, if so, how it became one and what kind of profession it is.

Definitions

Professionals are (usually full time) providers of expert services based on a knowledge of underlying principles. They have earned the right to recruit, educate, and certify themselves by maintaining high standards of expertise, service, and ethics.

Although historically, and still for many people, self certification—often with governmental approval (as for doctors and lawyers)—is the prime characteristic of a profession, the definition reaches beyond this to less easily defined but no less important areas.

Editors are . . . What *are* editors? 'Editor' does not yet have a clearly defined meaning. Traditionally, editors have been responsible for gathering, selecting, printing, and distributing scholarly articles for the profession. But today, although '*the* editor' of a particular journal is well understood to mean the scientific or medical editor who sets policy and directs its execution, '*an* editor' of a scientific periodical may only signify someone who is involved somehow in its production. Thus an editor may be a scientific or medical editor, a managing editor, a production editor, a copy editor, a letters editor, a regional editor, a statistical assistant, a board member, etc, etc. A relatively new term, 'author's editor', has come to mean someone who assists research scientists in writing articles or one who ghostwrites by converting raw data and a research protocol into a manuscript.

The diffusion and dilution of the term, based on its original prestige, and the aspirations of other workers are primary concerns of this chapter. In the discussion that follows I shall draw heavily on the writings of William J Goode, who has elaborated the characteristics of professions, and of Thomas Haskell, who focused on the conditions in which certain occupations became professionalised.

GOODE'S 'COMMUNITY'

One of the most compelling definitions of a profession is found in William J Goode's 'community within a community'.[4] He describes professions as contained communities in terms of their relations to the larger social structure in which they are embedded:

'(1) Its members are bound by a sense of identity.

(2) Once in it, few leave, so that it is a terminal or continuing status for the most part.

(3) Its members share values in common.

(4) Its role definitions *vis-à-vis* both members and non-members are agreed upon and are the same for all the members.

(5) Within the areas of communal action there is a common language which is understood only partially by outsiders.

(6) The community has power over its members.

(7) Its limits are reasonably clear, though they are not physical and geographical, but social.

(8) Though it does not produce the next generation biologically, it does so socially through its control over the selection of professional trainees, and through its training processes it sends these recruits through an adult socialisation process. Of course, professions vary in the degree to which they are communities, and it is not novel to view them as such.'[4]

GOODE'S DEFINITION AND MEDICINE

Goode's proposal clearly stands up well to perceptions of medicine. But clearly any model of professions, to be credible, *must* fit medicine, as it is one of the classic three that define the whole notion of profession. Medical doctors recognise their community, rarely leave it voluntarily, and for the most part share values that can be (and often are) enforced by the profession. Both the profession and the larger group understand what doctors are supposed to do, although insiders express it in a language that is often arcane to outsiders. Doctors (and their patients) understand that there are jobs that doctors will not and cannot do. And the public knows that when their family doctor retires, a suitable successor will show up in the office, trained, examined, and certified by other doctors in whom they place a kind of institutional trust.

Let us explore the extent to which Goode's model can be extended to include successively smaller communities, each contained in a larger like a set of Russian dolls. Biomedical research is proposed as the first test case: a community within 'a community within a community'. And then medical editors as an emerging community within biomedical research. Each then becomes a profession within a profession, with obligations to its most proximate reference group and to the larger communities that embrace it.

Let us first review Goode's criteria to see if scientists engaged in biomedical research fit the model regarding their surrounding community: medicine. Researchers who extend knowledge now play an especially important part in defining the traditional profession of medicine. They validate and extend the scientific basis of medical expertise that legitimates what doctors do and mandates what they should do. Furthermore, because a record of published research has become a major factor in appointing and promoting the faculty of most medical schools, researchers also appreciably influence the education and the orientation of practicing doctors. Their impact on the containing community is profound and continual. On a point by point basis:

(1) Biomedical researchers have a clear sense of identity within their specialty. They are expected to understand the principles and the craft of research beyond the basic knowledge of medicine that is understood by the surrounding community of doctors. Biomedical scientists work in a large variety of medical institutions, but most see their principal ties to research colleagues in their specialty in other institutions. They are linked by the exchange of research materials, ideas, data, and credit such as citations and acknowledgements. Together they attend scientific meetings that non-researchers rarely attend. They also frequent small invitational conferences and symposia that are restricted to specialists. Professional groups such as The Society for Clinical Investigation have ritualised selection processes and confer considerable prestige on their members.

Researchers see themselves as pursuing biomedical knowledge for its own sake and do not want to be bound to promises for practical outcomes, but they acknowledge that public support depends on the prestige and nobility of medicine as a healing profession. They thrive within the medical community more naturally and more logically than within the larger, balkanised community of research scientists in general. Citation data show the mutual citation of major medical journals and of biomedical research journals by the best general medical journals.

(2) Having chosen a career in biomedical research few leave it voluntarily, even though for most scientists with medical degrees there is a ready path to a lucrative career in medical practice. Many academic doctors pursue joint careers in practice and research (also see point (4) below). Failure to be promoted at academic institutions or to get grants or contracts to pursue research stand out as relatively common reasons for leaving the academy to join the larger community. Misconduct in research is a well publicised through rarer reason.

(3) In the past the values of the research community were rarely articulated, but the heroes of medical research (even if some stories were overly dramatic) served to reinforce its ideals. Biographies,

39

autobiographies, and histories of discoveries also reinforced high ideals. Peter Medawar's *Advice to a Young Scientist* and *Memoirs of a Thinking Radish* and Lewis Thomas' *Lives of a Cell* provide joyful excursions into the idealised (but still real) inquiring spirit of science.

More formal standards are set by editors and peer reviewers and increasingly by organisations like the Association of American Medical Colleges, the Institute of Medicine (USA), and the Royal College of Physicians; but until recently there were very few explicit, written codes of conduct for researchers.

Widely accepted values were too obvious to articulate: for instance, that science is devoted to truth. Recent episodes of sharp practices in research, especially those in biomedicine, have stimulated scientists to reaffirm that *as professionals* their relationships to each other and to the public are and must be based on high standards of truthfulness and trust. New knowledge and reliable processes for acquiring knowledge are their sole products and the *only* justification for public support.

(4) The distinctions between biomedical researchers and their surrounding community of doctors are more complicated than those that Goode has drawn for other professions. For instance, some researchers in academic medical centres hold a PhD degree and cannot practise medicine; and, whereas some MD biomedical researchers have given up all direct responsibility for patients, others continue to have clinical responsibilities. In some institutions, full time research faculty members and those clinical researchers who also see patients regard each other with suspicion and jealousy. Controversies have centred on criteria for promotion, the rate of advancement in rank, teaching responsibilities, the ability to get research grants and contracts, and the importance of clinical fees to some departmental budgets.

(5) Biomedical scientists share a rapidly changing technical vocabulary of their own; the private languages of science reflect expertise that identifies specialties and specialists. Furthermore, the rhetoric implicit in the structure of scientific articles helps to authenticate the published research for fellow researchers and for medical practitioners.

(6) The biomedical community exerts several kinds of power over its members. The most consequential is the mutually exercised power of the purse: peer review of grant and contract applications determine who shall be funded to continue research. As proved ability to get grants is frequently a criterion for university positions, peer

review has additional importance because of its effect on professional education. Applicants for grants and contracts must also provide a 'track record' of published articles to show that they are capable of carrying out the proposed research. Fellow scientists, acting as peer reviewers, control each other's opportunities in this process.

(7) The limits of the research community are primarily established by institutional affiliations. Biomedical researchers are most often identified with academic medical centres, satellite hospitals, independent research institutions, or pharmaceutical companies (and, increasingly, with more than one) or with new research institutions that straddle the boundaries between universities and industry.

(8) Biomedical researchers recruit and train the next generation of scientists. The research group also 'controls admission to training and requires far more education from its trainees than the containing community demands.'[4] Within certain academic medical communities, top researchers enjoy as much or more prestige than prominent clinicians, although full time scientists generally do not enjoy higher incomes. But it is increasingly difficult to find prominent clinicians who do not conduct some research. Medical schools are often ranked by the quality of research as much as or more than, by the quality of training and clinical practice.

The profound impact of biomedical science on the practice of medicine leads directly to the question of how that influence is conveyed to the profession at large.[6] Medical journals play the dominant role in mediating that influence. Their editors preside over the complicated present and the future of medical practice in a crucial fashion.

Social origins of professionalism

Before exploring medical editing as another community within a community, I should like to introduce Thomas Haskell's perspectives on the conditions under which society turns over certain specific responsibilities to groups that, as a result, declare themselves to be professions and take control of those duties. In describing the emergence of professional social science in the nineteenth century, Haskell has argued that the complexity of social problems and the consequent inability of ordinary people to predict and deal with factors beyond their control gave impetus to transferring problems from individuals and their families to a distinct group whose expertise qualified them to understand and deal with problems.

41

Their expertise developed in response to the challenge of the responsibility and then warranted even more authority and influence being transferred to them. Specialists agreed to divide problems among themselves so that each could develop the necessary skills.[7] Haskell accepts a concise notion of professionalism similar to Barber's.[8] In summary, the understanding required to perform certain important specialised tasks is accumulated and vouchsafed to certain conscientious individuals so that experience can improve their capacity to intervene effectively as professional caretakers of those tasks.

Wilensky, similarly, analysed the attempts of many occupations to become professional and set the following criteria: 'Any occupation wishing to exercise professional authority must find a technical basis for it, assert an exclusive jurisdiction, link both skill and jurisdiction to standards of training, and convince the public that its services are uniquely trustworthy.' And further, 'The service ideal is the pivot around which the moral claim to professional status revolves.'[9]

The editors of early journals

An appraisal of editors' roles in the past can add to our understanding of their work today. Furthermore, given Haskell's view of professionalism, we can assess to what extent scientific editing has changed over time, creating new complexities that have demanded more specialised (that is professional) skills to cope with new challenges.

Medical journals as we know them today have a mixed parentage. By considering the tasks and attitudes of editors of precursors to today's journals, we can begin to answer the question of whether or not editors are becoming more professional. Contributing to 'the common stock of medical knowledge' has been recognised as a professional obligation for at least 100 years. Thus publication in medical journals is traditionally important not only to teach doctors what is currently known, but to increase the store of information on which practice is based.

Of the two precursors of medical journals, medical magazines that flourished in the nineteenth century were essentially the property (and often the passion) of single individuals. Their views of what their colleagues needed to know competed in importance with the opportunity that publishing gave these gentlemen to disseminate their personal views of medical practice and to advertise medically relevant products. The other precursor was the correspondence of the secretaries of scientific societies in the seventeenth century that became the journals that reported observations and results of experiments of their members and correspondents.[10-12]

When the *British Medical Journal* (*BMJ*) began its new series in 1861, it did so over the objections that a journal sponsored by a public medical association would interfere with commercial publishing and with trade. The editor, William O Markham, used this very objection to justify the journal's role. 'A Journal which represents no individual interests, which is swayed by no party feeling, which has no commercial considerations to fetter its expressions or qualify its views—is surely a desirable medium for medical intercourse.'[13] He expressed his trust that 'the Journal will continue to be, as it always has been, a faithful exponent of those higher sentiments and feelings which, apart from the mere science and practice of the Profession, are necessary to give grace and credit to our vocation . . . In its very existence, it possesses a code of ethics, and by its authority enforces the recognition upon the Profession at large.'[13]

Even critics testified to the importance of editors. The *Medical Times and Gazette* (London) took the opportunity in an acid editorial to criticise the *former* editor for 'lively articles . . . wondrously curious to the popular mind and pleasant reading to all, [that] were incompatible with a due attention to the weightier matters of pathology and therapeutics.'[14] The new editor is characterised as being 'a hard working and rising physician.'[14]

The transition took place at a time when there was a great deal of turmoil about the professionalisation of medicine itself. Arguments about credentialising doctors focused on the competition between the university and the 'extra-academical school' in Edinburgh. The issues were those of autonomy, responsibility, expertise, and control.[15] Journals faced similar pressures and the *BMJ* asserted its determination to promote 'the science of medicine without truckling or pandering to the individual fancies either of the profession or the public.'[16] These goals were not then and are not now easy to achieve. In his discussion of the literature and the institutions of medicine at the time of America's first centennial, John Shaw Billings had little faith in medical editors' abilities to tackle these problems, although he acknowledged the importance of medical journals and his hopes for their improvement. 'Medical journalism is not a profession in this country. With one or two exceptions, our medical editors are engaged in practice and lecturing, and their labour in connection with the journals is not directly remunerative, nor is it the main object of their thoughts.'[17]

In the introductory essay to the first issue of the *Journal of Clinical Investigation* its editor, Alfred E Cohn, set a visionary tone for a scientific future of medicine as he associated the journal with the recent self consciousness of American medicine and the founding of university clinics oriented towards an increase in knowledge.[18]

Editors' organisations

If one of the marks of a profession is self consciousness, it is clear that editors of scientific journals early on recognised what they had in common with each other as well as their boldly stated differences. They recognised that there was strength in identifying themselves as editors and sharing views. In 1906, 125 medical editors attended the 37th annual meeting of the American Medical Editors Association (AMEA) at the Copley Square Hotel, Boston. The proceedings of that meeting include their constitution and bylaws. They discussed 'the relation of official and independent medical journalism and proper and improper medical advertisement'.[19] The final paper by James Evelyn Pilcher, the editor of the *Proceedings*, is an appraisal of his fellow editors and their weaknesses and strengths.[20] It divides medical editing into four classes of increasing degrees of qualification or professionalism. He speaks of the second class: 'While this may possibly be self-interest clothed in the garb of charity and generosity, the results, so far as the profession is concerned, are the same; the doctor gets much of value intermingled with some rather prejudiced information, but on the whole is greatly the gainer by his investment in this class of journalism'.[20] But he reserves his highest praise for the fourth class of medical editors who 'devote their entire time to the work'. He speaks of the incessant literary labour required for the 'constant supervision of the teeming mass of the new literature.' He argues for full time devotion to medical editing—'the medical journalism of the twentieth century increasingly demands the whole intellectual and physical energy of its editorial conductors, in the presence of the great aggregation of professional atoms which is daily falling upon the professional field to be excavated and investigated, and the clearing away of which, for the benefit of the twentieth century practitioner, will demand the entire absorption of the mind, soul and body of the conscientious medical editor, who really desires to be a helper to the profession, and a leader in the medical work of age.'[20] In short, a plea for professionalism.

In 1913, the AMEA published the first issue of a real journal—to succeed the *Proceedings*. The concerns expressed in that issue were quintessentially professional: (a) anonymous versus personal journalism, (b) inflated and unsubstantiated praise for medical remedies, (c) commercialism and medical advertising, and (d) professional relations.[21]

Modern pressures on editors and Haskell's criteria for professionalisation

No one can doubt that the conduct and the publication of research have become infinitely more complex in recent years, and that the need for a professional cadre to manage the problems is more imperative than ever before.[22–24] Thomas Stossel, former editor of the *Journal of Clinical Investigation*, among many others has recounted some of these changes in the research community.[23] They include the blurring of the distinction between basic and clinical research, the intense competitiveness of biomedical scientists, and, consequently, new demands put on editors who find themselves negotiating with authors about criteria for accepting submitted manuscripts. Complications are also caused by commercialism, new technologies, and international issues.

PEER REVIEW

Some criticisms of journals have focused on peer review. Editors have become active in promoting clarification and wider understanding of peer review, even though *editorial* peer review is only one aspect of a practice that has widespread ramifications for science policy.[25] [26] [27]

The utilisation of peer review is, in many ways, a much more complex and challenging task than the evaluation of manuscripts themselves (which, in any case, remains the editors' ultimate responsibility). It requires that the editor evaluate the reviewers as well as the manuscripts and also consider the social context of specialties, the standards of research institutions, and the impact of publication on funding patterns. Furthermore, peer review vastly increases the complexity of decisions by putting more specialised information at the disposal of the editor. In the past, no one expected editors to be expert at everything their journals published, but now specialist reviewers present such information, and expect the editors to consider and decide on the basis of extremely specialised knowledge. The process gives editors a greater arsenal of expert arguments; but it also leaves them more vulnerable to charges of unfairness in choosing or appraising reviewers' opinions. The editor's moral burden is also increased because confidentiality protects the identity of reviewers, while allowing the editor to share responsibility with unknown (presumably qualified) others. 'There is often ample evidence for both publishing and not publishing a manuscript, so the editor is free to choose almost any action within the broad confines established by the reviews, using the arguments available in the referees' reports as justification.'[26]

There is an even greater demand for discretion as editors know more and more secrets of the profession at just the time when the public seeks 'blue sky' reassurances about quality control mechanisms in science. Editors have successfully resisted attempts to rupture the confidentiality of the review process (Huth E, personal communication, 1990).[27–27b] Bombarded with inquiries from the press, the legislators, and even sociologists, they are often constrained by the rules of the game from disclosing news that would damage the profession. As a result, they can sound naive and self serving as they defend their craft.

AUTHORSHIP PRACTICES

Authorship practices are noticeably more complicated than they were only decades ago. Team research is a fact of life in modern science because of technological advances and increased specialisation as well as the growth of science. Increasing numbers of authors per submitted manuscript, and the fact that manuscripts are frequently submitted from more than one institution, often in more than one country, pose logistical and management problems. Authors are demanding speedier publication. At a time when the public and funding agencies are looking to journals for more direct accountability, the authors themselves are more numerous and more dispersed. There is increasing evidence of disputes among authors, dubious authorship, and proof that charlatans have named their colleagues as co-authors without ever consulting them.[28 28a] Authors revise and resubmit articles more often, which adds to the editors' burden as authors who once argued may change their minds and abdicate responsibility. Long before the International Committee of Medical Journal Editors proposed guidelines for authorship, several editors were debating their role in promoting responsible authorship practices.[2]

Editors are caught in a maelstrom of conflicting values. The emphasis on publication as a central criterion for allocating funding and for determining promotion and tenure in academic institutions was partly derived from a wish to utilise impartial judgements that were more fair than traditional networks. And yet other factors in the growth and complexity of science argue for judgements based on personal knowledge.[29]

THE SENSE OF URGENCY

Although it is a fact of modern life, some important things suffer from being rushed. Love and art come to mind, editing may be another. 'Editors are sometimes under pressure to publish articles rapidly and may, on occasion, short circuit their traditional review processes'.[30] And, on the other hand, 'some editors do not receive enough manuscripts and may promise acceptance without review of public talks'.[30] A serious professional challenge today may be to reduce the hurry and the worry. 'Editors have faced their limitations in situations where they have failed to accept seminal articles whose importance was evident in hindsight.'[2]

ARBITERS OF PROFESSIONAL MORALITY

There are few moral issues in medicine about which someone has not turned to medical editors to *do* something: express or reinforce a point of view, detect and identify offenders, and even censure transgressors. In the division of moral labour, editors currently are assigned a lion's share of the responsibility.[31] [32]

Marcia Angell has pointed out how editorial requirements can reduce the more common forms of deception in scientic publishing, such as fragmentation, 'loose' authorship, duplicate publication, and selection of data.[32] Although rejecting the notion that editors can always prevent egregious fraud such as plagiarism or fabrication of data, she proposes serious obligations for editors when they are made aware of the publication of fraudulent research.

Although they protest that they need to be able to, editors have found that they cannot rely absolutely on the integrity of the authors who submit manuscripts (Miller L. *Ethics of dual publication*. Talk given at 'Scholarly communication around the world', Philadelphia, 1983; unpublished observation.) They have had to make instructions to authors more explicit and detailed. They have also had to follow up reviewers' comments, asking questions about the smallest publishable fraction, about potential conflicts of interest, and about included and excluded authors. They are increasingly expected to enforce standards about preserving and sharing data, software, and research materials.

47

COMMERCIAL PRESSURE

Pharmaceutical companies have begun advertising ethical products direct to the public. This not only puts pressure on the financial basis of professional publishing, but means that the boundaries between publishing for doctors and for the public are increasingly less sharp. Widespread reporting of the substance of medical journal articles in the popular media is another challenge to editors. One approach has been to place an embargo on media reports, which itself draws criticism.[33] [34] [35] Other editors take the initiative and themselves prepare versions of articles for public presentation in print or on television.

As scientists are increasingly involved with work that affects corporate profits, editors have outlined new guidelines and requirements for disclosure of possible conflicts of interest.[35a] [35b]

PUBLICATION OF UNETHICAL RESEARCH

Editors have been torn by conflicting values in situations where they have been called on to publish reports of research based on unethical practices, but which have potential importance for medicine (Woodford FP, personal communication, 1984).[2] [36] [37]

STYLE AND SUBSTANCE IN SCIENTIFIC WRITING

Editors not only have their own personal styles but are in a position to, and often do, influence the style of individual authors and, cumulatively, of scientific writing as a whole. There are two schools of thought on this matter. The first is that a certain variety of style in a journal reflects important and pleasant differences among individual contributors. For instance, the *Biochemical Journal* in 1977 encouraged authors to employ their own style.[38] Other editors prefer a coherent style and are prepared to reject, correct, and even reconstruct submitted manuscripts to maintain this style. In the name of uniformity, there have been some stultifying excesses of impersonality in scientific writing. Editors and writers alike now welcome simple first person sentences in the active voice. O'Connor recommends a 'discreetly interventionist approach' as a compromise.[39]

STANDARDISATION OF REFERENCE STYLES

Some issues that editors face appear to be purely mechanical, but on consideration they prove to have consequences for scientific publishing. The standardisation of reference styles is one. Harvard style versus sequentially numbered references can raise pulses and voices to an extent that would surprise neutral observers and many readers.[40–42]

Editors have concerned themselves with other issues that have important implications for practice: the accuracy of dosages; the use of keywords in titles; completeness of references; the utility of tables, graphs, and legends; and the felicity and correctness of language.

INTERNATIONALISM OF SCIENTIFIC PUBLICATIONS

Editors are also expected to serve the goals of internationalism in science by providing extra services to foreign language authors, although others are tempted to lower standards to accommodate scientists from developing countries. Editors who wish to encourage scientists from Third World countries find that they spend an inordinate amount of time on some of the submitted manuscripts, trying to make them understandable. Though editors and reviewers grouse about the tribulation of doing so, there is more than a hint of civic pride behind the complaint.

IMMINENT FUTURE

Scientific journal editing is now challenged by opportunities and problems associated with new, non-traditional means of communication such as electronic journals, microforums, etc. Electronic communication technologies will have an impact on scientific creativity, on current notions of intellectual property, on international information exchange, and on many editorial decisions.[43]

MUNDANE TASKS

Many or most of journal editors' duties are, in some sense, professionally sacred. Their professionalism is tied to expert judgement and confidentiality and has great consequences for authors, readers, publishers, and society. They are responsible for:

(1) Determining the overall philosophy of the journal and acting to enforce it by choosing manuscripts for publication.

(2) Maintaining the peer review system by choosing, training, and evaluating peer reviewers. Peer review is increasingly recognised as an important factor in science policy.[22]

(3) Addressing larger issues of professional and social concern, and representing the profession to the press and the public.

In addition, however, many editors must be responsible for more mundane activities, such as: deciding on advertising and economic policies; managing relations with publishers and sponsoring societies; hiring and firing staff in a complex employment environment; choosing acid free paper and congenial type and format; etc.

QUALITY CONTROL IN BIOMEDICAL PUBLICATION

As guardians of professional journals, editors not only judge and select individual articles, in the process they are also obliged to define criteria that designate what is and what is not a professional journal. The rapid growth in numbers and varieties of published materials that purport to be scientific journals is not in dispute. Eugene Garfield, whose Institute (actually a corporation) for Scientific Information has argued that there are not necessarily too many, presents a version of 'rely on market forces' to show up bad journals for what they are.[44] He argues that, as long as the most respected journals of science retain and improve standards of publication, others will be forced to follow or eventually fall into disrepute. His prediction requires that scientists and editors note the disreputable journals and help to make shabby efforts less profitable than reputable ones.

INFORMATION RETRIEVAL AND INDEXING

Responsible editors can, and do, participate in deciding which journals should be indexed by major libraries such as National Library of Medicine and by secondary services such as *Chemical Abstracts*, BIOSIS, *Science Citation Index*, and *Excerpta Medica*. Editors' groups have discussed the financial and ethical impact of the so called 'grey literature' and controlled circulation journals.

'ENCROACHMENT'

Goode points out that contending members of professions never displace one another because empirical tests show the superiority of one or the other. On the contrary, he states that such tests are, in the nature of things, unlikely to be conducted because it would indicate that each contender acknowledged the *higher* authority of some third party and furthermore that disputes are likely to occur in 'new and obscure areas of human knowledge', which are notoriously difficult to judge.[45]

Perhaps because the derivative traits of a profession—wealth, prestige, and power—have not been granted in abundance to medical editors, there is currently no stampede of competitors. Nevertheless, in their wisdom, editors have cooperated in sharpening the tools of their trade.

Conclusion

There is no shortage of complexities or challenges for today's medical editors. There are clearly established, though rarely expressed, traditions of autonomy, responsibility, and expertise. Editors' groups such as the European Association of Science Editors and the Council of Biology Editors have organised but, although medical editors contribute effectively to their programme, there is not yet a clear sense of community under the auspices of these organisations. Similarly, groups of editors meet at large medical meetings but are not yet an effective influence as a group. The work of the International Committee of Medical Journal Editors has been salutary and has achieved extraordinary acceptance, considering that it is in no way, and never was intended to be, a representative group. It has prevailed because of good sense and clear, if cautious, purposes. When professions have got into trouble recently, it has usually been because of a lack of public confidence that the service ideal will consistently prevail over the loyalty that members feel to each other. Medical editing as an emerging profession still retains the service ideal. And the lack of solidarity among medical editors may thus stand them in good stead with their surrounding communities.

1 Wilensky HL. The professionalization of everyone? *American Journal of Sociology* 1964;LXX:137–58
2 Neter E. Chairman's address: editorial responsibilities limited. *CBE Views* 1980;**3**:9.
3 Wilensky HL. The professionalization of everyone? *American Journal of Sociology* 1964;LXX:148.
4 Goode WJ. Community within a community: the professions, *American Sociological Review* 1957;**22**:194–200.
6 Rodman H. The moral responsibility of journal editors and referees. *American Sociologist* 1970;**5**:351–7.
7 Haskell, Thomas. *The emergence of professional social science in the nineteenth century.* Ithaca, New York: Cornell University Press, 1980.
8 Barber B. Control and responsibility in the powerful professions. *Political Science Quarterly* 1978–9;**93**:599–615.
9 Wilensky HL. The professionalization of everyone? *American Journal of Sociology* 1964;LXX:138.
10 Cassedy JH. The flourishing and character of early American medical journalism. *Journal of the History of Medicine and Allied Sciences* 1983;**38**.
11 Burnham JC. The evolution of editorial peer review. *JAMA* 1990;**263**(10):1323.
12 McKie D. The scientific periodical from 1665 to 1798. *Philosophical Magazine* 1948;(commemoration issue):122–32.
13 Anonymous. The new series of the journal [editorial]. *Br Med J* 1861;i:14.
14 Anonymous. Association journalism [editorial]. *Medical Times and Gazette* (London) 1861; 2 Feb:118.
15 Anonymous. The battle of the colleges and the university. *Br Med J* 1861;i:66.
16 Anonymous. The medical times: a moral. *BMJ* 1861;i:146.

17 Billings JS. Literature and institutions. In: *A century of American medicine.* Philadelphia:Lea, 1876.

18 Cohn AE. Purposes in medical research. *J Clin Invest* 1925;**1**:1.

19 Pilcher JE, ed. Thirty seventh annual meeting. *Proceedings of the American Medical Editors Association* 1906; **37**:1–63.

20 Pilcher JE. The profession of medical journalism. *Proceedings of the American Medical Editors Association* 1906; **37**:58–63.

21 *Journal of American Medical Editors Association* 1913;**1**:41.

22 LaFollette MC. Journal peer review and public policy. *Science, Technology and Human Values* 1985;**10**:3–5. Cited in: Chubin DE, Hackett EJ. *Peerless science.* New York: State University of New York Press, 1990:4.

23 Stossel TP. Refinement in biomedical communication: a case study. *Science, Technology and Human Values* 1985;**10**:39.

24 Golley FB. Ethics in publishing. *CBE Views* 1981;**4**:26.

25 Lock SP. *A difficult balance: editorial peer review in medicine.* London: Nuffield Provincial Hospitals Trust, 1985. Reprinted London: BMJ, 1991.

26 Chubin DE, Hackett EJ. *Peerless science.* New York: State University of New York Press, 1990:89.

27 Guarding the guardians: research on editorial peer review. *JAMA* 1990;**263**:1309–1456 (entire issue).

27a Lundberg GD. 'It's over, Debbie' and the euthanasia debate. *Jama* 1988;**259**:2142.

27b Lundberg GD. Editorial freedom and integrity. *JAMA* 1988;**260**:2563.

28 Peters RM. Scientific responsibility in medical reporting [letter]. *Ann Thorac Surg* 1988;**46**:377.

28a Kennedy D. *Academic authorship. Memorandum to the Faculty of Stanford University, 1985.* Palo Alto, California: Stanford University, 1985.

29 Stossel TP. Volume: papers and academic promotion. *Ann Intern Med* 1987;**106**:146.

30 Stossel TP. Speed. *N Engl J Med* 1985;**313**:123.

31 Benichoux R. Politicians and scientific fraud: spectators or actors? *Earth & Life Science Editing* 1984;**23**:3.

32 Angell M. Editors and fraud. *CBE Views* 1983;**6**:3.

33 Ingelfinger F. Medical literature: the campus without the tumult. *Science* 1970;**170**:831.

34 Relman AS. More on the Ingelfinger rule. *N Engl J Med* 1988;**318**:1125–6.

35 Silber F. Medical editors' dilemma. *Science* 1970;**170**:388.

35a Lundberg GD, Flanagin A. New requirements from authors: signed statements of authorship responsibility and financial disclosure. *JAMA* 1989;**262**:2003–4.

35b Relman AS. Economic incentive in clinical investigation. *N Engl J Med* 1989;**320**:933–4.

36 Brackhill Y, Hellegers AE. Ethics and editors. *Hastings Cent Rep* 1980;**10**:20–4.

37 Woodford FP. Ethical experimentation and the author. *N Engl J Med* 1972;**286**:892.

38 Editorial Board. Policy of the journal and instructions to authors: amendments. *Biochem J* 1977;**161**:1–2.

39 O'Connor M. *Editing scientific books and journals.* Tunbridge Wells: Pitman Medical, 1978:50.

40 Henning M. More on the Harvard style [letter]. *CBE Views* 1983;**6**:2.

41 International Committee of Medical Journal Editors. Uniform requirements for manuscripts submitted to biomedical journals. *BMJ* 1991;**302**:338–41.

42 O'Connor M. Standardisation of bibliographical reference systems. *Br Med J* 1978;i:31–2.

43 *Toward the year 2000: new forces in publishing.* Gutersloh, Germany: Bertelsmann Foundation Publishers, 1989.

44 Garfield E. [Letter to the editor.] *Bioscience* 1983;**33**:76–7.

45 Goode WJ. Encroachment, charlatanism and the emerging profession: psychology, sociology and medicine. *American Sociological Review* 1960;**25**:902.

PART 2
THE POINTS OF VIEW

About editors

A RELMAN

I write this chapter shortly after having announced that I will retire from my present position next year. The occasion stimulates reflection not only about my own career, but about the editor's profession in general. What follows are some observations about editing and editors, based largely on my own experiences as editor of two medical journals: the *Journal of Clinical Investigation* (1962–67) and the *New England Journal of Medicine* (1977–91)

Although they reflect personal experience, these comments are not autobiographical, at least not intentionally. I intend rather to discuss broad issues of concern to all those interested in how medical journals function. I will focus on the role of editors and how they do their job. I will also consider the training and background of editors and the present status and future prospects of the medical editing profession.

I shall imagine that I am being interviewed by the search committee for my successor. Because some committee members have had little or no direct contact with medical editing they are seeking background information before turning to the task of selecting a candidate.

Committee: Dr Relman, what are the responsibilities of the editor of a journal like the *New England Journal of Medicine*?

ASR: The editor establishes the journal's standards and editorial policies. She* is directly responsible for the quality and style of the journal and ultimately for the selection of its content, but is only indirectly responsible for the substance of the journal's content.

Committee: The editor is the chief executive officer of the editorial

---

* Editing, like most other professions, is becoming increasingly epicene. Four recent appointees to important general medical editorial posts have been women. In arbitrarily choosing the feminine pronoun my purpose is simply to avoid awkward 'he or she' circumlocutions, not to imply that either sex has a monopoly on qualifications for journal editorship.

office; why do you quality her responsibility for the journal's content?

ASR: The editor makes (or at least oversees) the final decision as to what is published and how it is revised and edited before publication but, except for material she personally writes and signs, she cannot and should not be fully accountable for what is written in the journal. That responsibility rests in all cases with the authors. Just as editors cannot take personal credit for the ideas and research results presented by others, so they cannot be held personally responsible for defects in that material discoverable only in retrospect. On the other hand, editors are responsible for the quality of the review process and therefore are accountable for deficiencies that could reasonably have been identified before publication.

Committee: What role should the editor of a peer reviewed journal play in the selection of material for publication?

ASR: A useful way to look at the editor's role is in terms of its activity or passivity. At one end of such a spectrum is the largely 'passive' editor who sees herself simply as a facilitator and administrator of the review process and therefore leaves the selection of manuscripts largely in the hands of the referees. Split decisions are resolved by soliciting additional opinions to clarify the disputed issues and then tallying the referees' votes. This kind of editorship is most likely to be found in specialist journals, when editors serve only on a part time basis and have no time for greater involvement and when selection of articles depends largely on scientific considerations with which the referees are most familiar. Editorial management of this sort makes for an essentially technical journal with no consistent character or style and little appeal to readers outside a narrow specialty.

Journals with a broader range and variety of content usually require a different editorial philosophy and more input from the editor. There are many competing claims for space in the general journal, which can be resolved successfully only by a fully engaged editor who has a clear sense of what her readers want and what the journal ought to be. General medical journals like the *New England Journal of Medicine* publish not only clinical research studies but reviews, commentary, letters, and a wide range of articles dealing with the social, economic, legal, ethical, and historical aspects of medicine. The editor of such a journal needs to be much closer to the 'active' end of the spectrum. She knows that her readers represent a diversity of medical interests and specialties, so she must select research articles that have the broadest appeal and can be read and understood by readers with diverse backgrounds. Regarding the research articles, scientific soundness, as judged by the referees, is a necessary but not sufficient condition for acceptance. Timeliness, originality, readability, and the journal's need for a balanced mix of subject material are also important, and these concerns must be weighed by the editor and her staff. As for the rest of the general journal's content—the reviews and commentary and all the articles on more general subjects—the editor's role here is even more crucial because outside referees, although often able to give helpful advice, are not likely to have the broad overview or the sense of the journal's character and purpose that the in house editorial staff bring to their task. Even if referees do have their own views on these matters, they are rarely unanimous and not infrequently at odds with those of the editor. Whereas differences of opinion about the technical merits of a scientific contribution can usually be resolved by seeking additional expert advice, differences of opinion about matters of taste and judgement must be settled at the editor's desk, where ultimate responsibility for the journal's policies resides.

Committee: If the editor of the *New England Journal of Medicine* plays such a pivotal role in the selection of material, isn't there a danger that the articles and letters of opinion will be slanted toward the editor's own views and that the journal's table of contents will reflect her personal interests?

ASR: There is that possibility, so the editor must take great care to see that the journal's opinion pages and correspondence section are open to all points of view and that the selection of articles reflects the broad interests of the journal's readers. She should be free to express her own opinions from time to time in signed editorials, but her primary function is to act as the honest and impartial moderator of an open forum. On the other hand, the editor's personal influence on the general style and character of the journal is important, for without firm guidance a journal easily becomes amorphous and dull. Of course, a wise editor leans heavily on the advice of staff, but even the most competent and experienced of staffs will sometimes be divided on difficult problems of editorial judgement, leaving the final decision to the editor.

Committee: It sounds as if the editor has a heavy burden of responsibility. What kind of training is needed?

ASR: There are no schools for medical editors. They learn their craft mainly through experience. There are many paths to the editor's desk and no prescribed course of training or professional certification is required to get there. However, most future editors will have evinced an early interest in the topic by their association with a medical journal as a reviewer and a member of an editorial board or part time editorial staff. Some serve apprenticeships as associate or deputy editors before assuming senior responsibility.

In any case, I believe that the essential editorial abilities are innate, not learned. The technical skills of editing can be acquired but the qualities of mind and temperament necessary for success cannot.

Committee: What are the qualities we should look for?

ASR: Outstanding editors are characterised by intelligence, integrity, good critical judgement, and a sense of humour. They also have an ear for language and an ability to appreciate and write clear, graceful prose. I suppose the latter can be learned to a degree, but the other traits are inherent. Editing is a generous ministering profession, like the practice of medicine, so editors should also be unselfish. They should be interested in the ideas and the work of others, and they should be able to get satisfaction from working with authors to improve their papers.

Perhaps the most important qualities of all are moral courage and a sense of fair play. Editors are constantly being called on to make difficult judgements and to resolve disputes in a manner that all parties will respect even when disagreeing with the result. Their decisions may have important consequences for friends, influential people, businesses, or the public, and they must have the courage to do what they think is right regardless of how uncomfortable it may be. This requires editorial independence.

Committee: Your mention of independence raises the subject of the relation between the editor and the journal's owners. What should be the terms?

ASR: Owners are owners, and they have the legal right to run their journal as they wish, but if they own a peer reviewed professional journal and they want it to be respected and trusted, they should not interfere with its editorial management. They should not attempt to influence the editor's choice of content, or to control the opinion expressed by authors. To do so would cast doubt on the journal's integrity—scientific and otherwise. The separation between the political and economic interests of the owners and the editorial management should be clear and unquestioned. For example: (a) advertisers should have no influence on the editor's decisions, and no privileged access to her office; and (b) the opinion pages of the journal should not favour the political or economic positions held by the owners, but should be open to all points of view. A peer reviewed general medical journal has a different standing from the usual newspaper or newsmagazine and its professional obligations require a different standard of editorial independence. It would not do for us to claim that most, *but not all*, of our content was independently selected by the editors, thus implying that the remainder was dictated or at least influenced by our owners' policies. Presumably we would at least want to say that the selection of all the scientific material was free from such influence, but that would not reassure our readers and, in any case, distinctions between what is 'scientific' and what is not tend to become blurred. Confidence in the independence and integrity of our editorial management, on which so much of our reputation depends, would be undermined. Furthermore, much of a general journal's appeal resides in its non-technical content; if the latter represented only the approved policies of the owners, reader interest would surely decline.

If all this is true then the editor of the medical journal should be insulated as much as possible against day to day pressures from her employers. The editor of a journal like ours can be compared to the music director of a major symphony orchestra. The trustees of the orchestra hire the music director and have the power to fire him (under terms usually defined contractually) but they do not interfere with his work. The director selects the members of the orchestra and the programmes they will play, and he is responsible for the quality of their performances. In the long run, if the trustees are not satisfied with the result or if the audiences and critics are not happy, the trustees can replace the director. But until that happens, the director is in charge.

Committee: Returning to editing as a career, are there organisations concerned with the medical editing profession and the cultivation of editorial skills?

ASR: The Council of Biology Editors and the European Association of Science Editors are the largest and most important. As their names suggest, however, their membership is not limited to medical editors; indeed, most members are not doctors and they work in many other scientific fields on a wide variety of publications. Membership is open to anyone interested in writing, editing, or publishing, not simply those with editorial responsibility for peer reviewed journals. These organisations serve an important function and many—but by no means all—medical editors are members. Yet their size and the diversity of their membership inevitably constrain their ability to concentrate on some of the problems unique to medicine and this limits their appeal to medical editors.

The International Committee of Medical Journal Editors—the so called 'Vancouver group'—is a much smaller and more selective organisation, consisting of a handful of editors representing the leading peer reviewed general medical journals that publish in England or use English summaries. This group has been very active in promulgating standards for editorial policies and practices that have gained worldwide acceptance among medical journals. However, it is essentially a senior editor's club, and its present small size precludes participation by junior staff members and by hundreds of other doctors who are part time editors of medical specialty journals.

In my opinion it may now be time for the Vancouver group to expand its membership or for a new organisation to be established that would be open to all editors of peer reviewed medical journals. I make 'peer reviewed' an essential qualification because it more or less clearly separates two classes of journals with widely disparate standards and objectives and therefore with different editorial needs.

Committee: Does the active, 'hands on' kind of editor you seem to be recommending as your successor have a long term future? Will electronic publishing make traditional editing obsolete? Can you foresee a time when new data will be made instantly available simply by entry into a computerised database, thus obviating the editor's role?

ASR: I think not. Editors serve a function that can only be facilitated by the computer, but not replaced by it. New data, before they become part of any database, must be peer reviewed if they are to be reliable, and editors will always be needed to manage the peer review process. However, even peer reviewed computerised databases will not meet the needs of general readers who want to browse through current publications to learn about interesting and important developments in many topics. Computerised databases are invaluable in searching for published reports and providing answers to specific questions, but they are of no help in selecting or evaluating the new developments that will be of interest to the general reader.

Whatever the electronic future of informatics may be, editorial supervision will always be needed for reviewing, selecting, editing, and interpreting scientific data and for the continuing effort to maintain and improve the quality of our information base. Beyond this, if general journals survive—and I believe they surely will—we will require editors to select and edit their varied content and to preside over the lively forum which only such journals can offer. That computers will play an increasingly important role in the processing, communication, and use of information, and in the technology of publishing, cannot be doubted, but we will always need the intellectual input of editors to help ensure the quality, interest, readability, and relevance of our information. So, as far as I can see, editors are not likely to become obsolete. Indeed, as new information is generated at a quickening pace, the editorial function will become increasingly critical. That being the case, identifying and encouraging editorial talent is more important than ever before. I wish you good luck with your task.

Pluralism please

ROBIN FOX

'When I divide the week's contributions into two piles—one that we are going to publish and the other that we are going to return—I wonder whether it would make any real difference to the journal or its readers if I exchanged one pile for the other.'[1] Perhaps if T F Fox had gone in for exclamation marks to label his jokes, this remark would not have been so widely quoted. In reality he took immense trouble over the selection of articles, and sought outside advice on many of them. There was, I confess, one occasion when a caseful of submitted articles blew off the car roof into the headwaters of the River Medway and the most mudstained items had to be accepted. Alas, the outcome of this random selection process was not recorded.

It is just three weeks ago (at the time of writing) that I took on the editorship of the *Lancet* and with it Stephen Lock's invitation to contribute to the meeting at Leeds Castle. I shall offer just a few observations on the way we choose papers for the *Lancet*—on how the procedure evolved under T F Fox's three successors—and then indicate some unease about the style in which we general medical journals present original material to our readers.

Selection

Taking over from my father in 1963, Ian Douglas-Wilson continued to seek advice on difficult papers but relied more on his nose for good science—and his nose was good. 'It has the "Colgate ring of confidence"' he would say, casting a paper without more ado into the basket for editing. By cutting the decision phase to 10 days or so and sharpening up editorial and printing operations, he was able to offer publication of full papers in three or four weeks, sometimes less. Authors found this service highly attractive, and the policy drew many new ones (and good papers) to the journal. The occasional disaster did not worry Douglas-Wilson at all: readers, he argued, would be put straight by observing the demolition process in the correspondence columns. His high risk strategy was in accord with the revolutionary spirit of the day and, when I arrived in 1968, was making the *Lancet* an exciting place to work in. Douglas-Wilson's view was that his system, relying heavily on the judgement of an independent editor, cut out the influence of envy, elitism, conservatism, and other banes. 'If an editor does not please himself', he used to say, 'he will not please anybody'.

None the less, when Ian Munro took the editorial chair in 1976, it was clear that the buccaneering approach had to end. In the USA, where the journal was now being printed locally, doctors were becoming reluctant even to cast an eye on research papers that did not bear the 'pass' sticker of peer review. So we decided that, thenceforth, papers must not be printed in the *Lancet* without first being scrutinised by one or more external advisers. My great regret is that, from 1976, we failed to mount a randomised trial to assess the impact of this exercise on the quality of what we printed. That it has made the scientific work that we publish less vulnerable to criticism I do not doubt; but I do have a feeling that it penalises non-conformists. (How we could have measured this I do not know.) In addition, the *Lancet* has certainly lost some of its competitive edge in timing, though we are still able to say no, if not yes, more quickly than many of our contemporaries. By concentrating peer review on the papers that appeal to the editorial staff we cut out much paperwork and delay.

What sort of papers are we looking for? Naturally, we are particularly keen to publish articles that will substantially advance clinical science or practice; but a glance at the general journals in any given week shows that the research community cannot keep pace even with the demands of the *Lancet*, the *New England Journal of Medicine*, the *British Medical Journal*, and the *Journal of the American Medical Association* (*JAMA*). Although we are offered more than 4000 papers a year, there are some weeks in which we are hard pressed to find a single paper in this category. Just one such article a week, in those four journals, would be 200-plus a year—a lot to ask of the medical community. Ken Warren has recorded that most of the important papers appear in just a few of the journals; such papers are scarce.

When I divide the week's contributions into two piles . . . I can expect about 80% in the no basket and 20% in the perhaps basket. On 20 July 1990 I looked at the fate of the first 100 received in that month. Seventy eight had already been declined, or were about to be so, after scrutiny by two or more of the editorial staff and subsequent discussion. The main reason for rejection was that they did not advance knowledge or would not influence practice (38%). Then came specialist interest only (22%), design defect (10%), and prematurity (5%). Of the remaining 22 papers, two had been accepted—an epidemiological article after peer review and an opinion piece without external review. About half the peer reviewed items are eventually published as full papers, and a few more are printed in the form of letters to the editor. This particular batch contained several items that had generated editorial enthusiasm, but only one (a large vaccine trial) that might represent a jump forward in clinical terms.

As I see it, the process of peer review has three functions—namely, to assess originality; to identify defects of design that make a work irremediably unpublishable; and to identify faults that can be corrected. My guess is that an increase in the number of external reviewers for each paper would increase the number of points on which we sought revisions, rather than the number of outright rejections. We now hope to assess, in a randomised study, the effect on our own operation of formal and separate statistical review. The question is, will this additional measure usefully add to the statistical evaluations supplied by our customary advisers (whom we sometimes encourage to consult statistician colleagues)? What should be the end point? And who should evaluate the result?

Presentation

A general journal should try to cover all important developments in medicine, and offer a platform for criticism and new ideas. I applaud the variety of ways this is achieved in the major weeklies—journals do have their own personalities. When we get beyond the formal reports we are in a world of free debate, almost a slice of medical life. But are editors agreeing too much about the way they present the formal reports—temples of knowledge erected on the shaky pillars of IMRAD (Introduction, Methods, Results, and Discussion)? Though a supporter of the Vancouver style, which must have spared several forests and thousands of secretarial working hours as well as providing much needed guidance on contentious matters, I fear that the International Committee of Medical Journal Editors (ICMJE), among others, may have helped to paint the reporting of science into a corner. At the pleasant gatherings of the ICMJE, our consensus adds increasingly to the detail and complexity we ask of our contributors within the structure of IMRAD. John Maddox remarked the other day that most contributors have an interest that 'what they say should be unassailable even at the cost that it is unintelligible'.[2] I say that editors, above all, should be resisting this trend. Defensive editing we do not need.

A couple of years ago the *Lancet* printed a very long article with a practical message about thrombolysis in myocardial infarction. The conclusions were of importance to many thousands of clinicians, but I wonder how many individuals read the paper from beginning to end (other than the authors, the referees, the printers, and me). A paper that is heavily cited may be read seldom. How can we declutter such articles so that they will be read avidly and critically over the toast and marmalade, and at the same time accommodate the legitimate demands of the statisticians, the molecular biologists, and the information scientists for ever more detail?

The main concerns of the ICMJE over the past decade have been references, authorship, duplicate publication, and fraud. The challenges for the next decade will surely be the conflict between information content and readability. Every so often, we hear the view that we need only a few journals, as much of the material is archival and could be stored and retrieved by electronic means. For general journals, perhaps the answer to our dilemma is to adopt *part* of this solution—to cut down on detail that, though of deep interest to some, would cause the average reader to switch off. After inspection by the editors and peer reviewers, the supplementary information would be stored by the journal for onward transmission. (The level of demand for such information would itself tell us something about the needs of the readers.)

General journals such as the *British Medical Journal*, *JAMA*, the *Lancet*, and the *New England Journal of Medicine* should detach themselves a little from the information industry and experiment, individually, with new ways. In correspondence and on the telephone, authors show wit and wisdom: why then are their articles so stiff and stilted? If the soul of wit is brevity, we might start there—by setting fiercer limits on length. What is the purpose of the reference list (it is no business of the journals to supply fodder for the citation analysts)? Why do we settle so often for IMRAD when we know that this structure encourages authors to deviate from the truth (given the chance, authors seem happy to tell 'how it really happened')?

Lastly, a word about the correspondence columns. No paper is unassailable, and a vigorous to and fro in the letters pages can be educational to bystanders as well as to authors. All journals should welcome critical correspondence; editors should encourage the notion that peer review continues after publication, and critical correspondence should be recorded by the information retrieval services.

I have suggested that general journals should behave rather differently from their specialist brethren. They should also avoid agreeing too much among themselves. Pluralism please.

1 Fox TF. *Crisis in communication: the functions and future of medical journals.* London: Athlone Press, 1965.
2 Maddox J. What to do with extraneous data. *Nature* 1990;**346**:215.

Whom do journal editors serve?

M ANGELL

Editors often find themselves dealing with competing claims. Claims of timeliness may compete with those of thoroughness, newsworthiness with caution, liveliness with sobriety, and so on. Long term interests often compete with more immediate interests. Should an editor publish a study that has important implications and is *probably* valid, when it is methodologically flawed and *may* not stand the test of time? Sometimes the competing claims are more personal. No one likes to say no to a friend, particularly if the friend is a respected senior investigator, but an editor must be willing to do so again and again. Or the claims may be political, as, for example, when authors oppose the positions of the professional society that owns the journal. And sometimes the competing claims touch on the very survival of the journal, as when advertisers demand that the journal's content reflects their interests. Obviously, an important attribute of a good editor is decisiveness. And a thick skin helps. But decisiveness alone is not enough. In addition, there needs to be a theoretical construct on which decisions are based—a construct that enables an editor to sort out the competing claims and weigh them. Without this, decisions may be contradictory, and decisiveness becomes caprice or stubbornness. I shall propose such a theoretical construct here.

In sorting out competing claims, it helps to think in terms of legitimacy. Who, in fact, has a legitimate claim on the editor's consideration and what is the nature of that claim? It is useful, I believe, to think of a medical journal as having four constituencies: the public, readers, authors, and owners. Usually the interests of these constituencies coincide, but sometimes they conflict and editors must choose among them. On what basis should editors make their choice? And what is the role of their own standards and

67

integrity, apart from the immediate interests of their consitituencies? I intend to discuss the claims of the four constituencies separately and argue that editors should in general honour them in the order discussed. Finally, I shall discuss the importance of the editor's own standards and of editorial independence.

The public

There is much rhetoric about the pubic's right to news of medical research. The public, after all, usually pays for the research and its health is at stake. In reality, however, the public interest is usually not a factor in editorial decisions about publication. Most biomedical research does not yield a conclusive answer that would warrant a change in medical advice or the way patients are treated. Instead, research usually suggests avenues for further research, which leads to changes only cumulatively. When a single study *does* have dramatic practical implications, it is usually all the more important to wait to make sure the results are confirmed before acting on them. Rhetoric tends to get ahead of reality, in part because the public does not fully understand the tentative nature of biomedical research (it prefers 'breakthroughs') and the popular media are competing for stories about medical research. It is important, I believe, that editors do not confuse the public welfare with the media's desire for stories; they are not the same.

Sometimes, however, a paper contains information of urgent practical significance. In those cases, editors must give the public interest first priority and cooperate in all efforts to get the information to the public. This means suspending strictures against prior publication or publicity before publication. The *New England Journal of Medicine*, for example, has a policy, known as the Ingelfinger rule,[1] of considering reports for publication only if their substance has not been published elsewhere. Most of the major journals have similar policies, and the International Committee of Medical Journal Editors has also gone on record as discouraging multiple reports of the same study.[2] We waive this policy for reports of immediate practical significance or of intense public concern. In these cases, prior publication of the results of a study does not preclude the journal considering a report based on the same work. In recent years such exemptions have usually concerned AIDS research, but not always. In May 1990 we published a report of the successful use of methylprednisolone to treat acute spinal cord injury,[3] and we waived the Ingelfinger rule, as well as the embargo on the use of stories from the journal by the popular media. Similarly, the rule was not applied to a recent study of isoprinosine for treating HIV infection,[4] or to two studies published in October 1990 reporting the efficacy of very low dose zidovudine for HIV infection.[5] [6] To be sure, there is a risk in encouraging researchers to present their findings direct to the media; the findings may later be found to be problematic or unwarranted in the review and revision process. This is the risk that leads us in general to discourage announcements of research results before publication, except for presentations at scientific meetings and abstracts of those meetings. Nevertheless, when research has clear and unequivocal implications for treatment or behaviour, editors must help to see that news of the results is disseminated. Usually we do this by expediting the review process; then, when we have some indication of the likely validity of the work, but before publication, we waive the Ingelfinger rule and the embargo. We also defer to the judgement of government health agencies, such as the National Institute of Health or the Centers for Disease Control, when they deem it necessary to publicise a study even before submission of a manuscript.

Readers

A successful journal—that is, a journal with many loyal subscribers—is almost by definition one with an editor who gives a very high priority to the claims of readers. Unless the journal is a small specialist journal with readers and authors being the same people, the interests of readers may differ greatly from those of authors. Just what are the obligations of editors to readers?[7] Obviously, they include selecting papers for publication on the basis of interest and importance to that particular readership. Research reports must be relevant and original, and other articles, including review articles, must in some way offer new insights that would interest the readership. Often editors must reject scientifically sound work because it doesn't meet these criteria. Equally important, editors must make sure that the level of presentation of reports they publish is appropriate. Readers should not regularly have to refer to other sources to understand papers, and readers of general journals should not have to struggle with specialised language. Frequently editors must ask for repeated revisions to make papers readable for their subscribers. Authors are often annoyed by what seems to them a trivial issue, but in this situation editors need to see themselves as advocates for their readers.

The most difficult obligation to readers is seeing that published papers are as scientifically valid as possible. This means thoroughly reviewing manuscripts to make certain that the design of the study was appropriate, the methods adequate, the results properly analysed, and the conclusions warranted by the data. Editors should ask for as many revisions as they, with the advice of their reviewers, think necessary. This iterative process of review and revision is often time consuming, and competes with the understandable desire of authors to have a speedy decision. There may thus be a tension between accuracy, which may loosely be considered to be an obligation to readers, and speed, which may be considered to be an obligation to authors (and sometimes to the media). I believe that both are important, but when they conflict accuracy is usually the more important.

Authors

A journal cannot survive long if researchers do not choose to submit manuscripts to it for publication. Whether they do so depends to a great extent on the quality and prestige of the journal, but it also depends on the way in which the editor treats the authors. Authors have a right to expect promptness in reaching a decision about their manuscripts, within the constraints imposed by the process of review and revision just described. They also have a right to expect courtesy and honesty. A manuscript usually represents a substantial investment of its authors' time, energy, and professional hopes, and editors should not dismiss this investment lightly. Although they cannot be expected to provide detailed reasons for all rejections, they should let authors know when the reason for rejection is primarily editorial rather than scientific, that is, when it concerns suitability for the particular journal. Scientific shortcomings, including reasons for rejection, are usually detailed in reviewers' comments for authors. Editors must make sure that the tone of these comments is respectful, especially if the work is being rejected. They should also be willing to reconsider decisions to reject papers if the authors believe that they can satisfactorily rebut the reviewers' criticism. Finally, it is important that editors are scrupulously fair in dealing with authors. They must not show favouritism towards certain authors or institutions, but should deal with each paper on its merits.

What claims of authors should editors not honour? Firstly, because of greater obligations to readers, editors should not compromise the editorial process to give authors a rapid decision. Authors are often greatly concerned about priority, and editors must be prepared to resist pressures to short circuit the process because of this. Secondly, editors must be willing to hold authors to the editorial standards of the journal, for the sake of their readers. This means that authors may not include all the supporting documentation they might wish, they may have to temper exuberant interpretations, shorten the presentation, and sacrifice their jargon. Accomplishing these changes may be difficult, and editors would do well to be open to rebuttal or compromise, but they should have foremost in mind the needs of their readers.

Owners

Editors are directly dependent on their journals' owners in the sense that their jobs depend on the owners. They serve at the owners' pleasure, and, unlike readers and authors, owners do not simply fade away one by one if they are dissatisfied. In a practical sense, then, owners would seem to be the most important constituency for editors to satisfy. Fortunately, the situation is more complicated. Very few owners of medical journals believe that they have the expertise to oversee the content and editorial processes of their journals, and they hire editors to do precisely that. In addition, there is a journalistic tradition of editorial independence, as well as the scientific necessity that research be judged by peers on its merits. All of this tends to mitigate the day to day claims of owners on editors. Nevertheless, journals differ in the degree of governance by their owners. Some have a tradition of complete editorial independence. Lesser degrees of independence can create severe problems for journal editors. For example, editors of journals owned by professional societies may feel pressure to publish papers by members of the society. Or journal owners may transmit to their editors pressures from advertisers to publish work favourable to their products or to suppress or play down unfavourable results. Editors should do everything possible to convince their owners that such pressures are not in their long term interests. Whatever the immediate gains, journals will not thrive unless their editors can serve their readers and contributors without undue political or economic concern.

Journals are more credible and interesting to readers when it is understood that their editors can accept or reject anything on its merits and can present all points of view. Furthermore, talented editors are difficult to recruit unless they are assured of substantial independence. Winning or maintaining editorial independence may be very difficult for editors acting alone, but acting in concert they can do much to bolster the principle. In 1988 the International Committee of Medical Journal Editors issued a statement on editorial freedom which affirmed the principle of editorial independence.[8] According to this statement, owners may appoint and dismiss editors, but they should not attempt to influence editorial content direct.

Editors are people too

An important, but underappreciated determinant of the decisions of editors are their own individual standards, which are often difficult to articulate but strongly held. Even when editors agree on an approach to their job and on a framework for making decisions, these individual standards lead to different types of decisions and to journals being very different from one another. They determine the threshold, for example, for turning down a paper of immediate or sensational interest to readers because of considerations of taste or fairness or because of persistent doubts about its validity. They also influence the topics covered by the journal and set its style. Such differences among editors add to the variety and interest of the various biomedical journals, and should therefore not be discouraged. Nevertheless, some degree of uniformity among editors and some consistency on the part of any one editor are desirable. Otherwise the editorial process becomes too vulnerable to the prejudices and idiosyncracies of editors, and we can lose sight of the primary educational goal of the enterprise. A construct such as I have described enables editors to analyse and adjudicate relatively objectively the many competing claims they face. It thus contributes to uniformity and consistency among editors without sacrificing personality. It also provides for individual editors a gauge against which they can measure their decisions so that over time they do not become too subjective or arbitrary. Editors need some ballast—particularly when they have been in the job for some time—and remembering whom they serve helps to provide it.

1 Relman AS. More on the Ingelfinger rule. *N Engl J Med* 1988;**318**:1125–6.
2 International Committee of Medical Journal Editors. Uniform requirements for manuscripts submitted to biomedical jurnals. *N Engl J Med* 1991;**324**:424–8.
3 Bracken MB, Shepard MJ, Collins WF, *et al*. A randomized, controlled trial of methylprednisolone or naloxone in the treatment of acute spinal-cord injury: results of the Second National Acute Spinal Cord Injury Study. *N Engl J Med* 1990;**322**:1405–11.
4 Pedersen C, Sandstrom E, Petersen CS, *et al*. The efficacy of inosine pranobex in preventing the acquired immunodeficiency syndrome in patients with human immunodeficiency virus infection. *N Engl J Med* 1990;**322**:1757–63.
5 Fischl MA, Parker CB, Pettinelli C, *et al*. A randomized controlled trial of a reduced daily dose of zidovudine in patients with the acquired immunodeficiency syndrome. *N Engl J Med* 1990;**323**:1009–14.
6 Collier AC, Bozzette S, Coombs RW, *et al*. A pilot study of low-dose zidovudine in human immunodeficiency virus infection. *N Engl J Med* 1990;**323**:1015–21.
7 Relman AS, Angell M. How good is peer review? *N Engl J Med* 1989;**321**:827–9.
8 Lundberg GD. Editorial freedom and integrity. *JAMA* 1988;**260**:2563.

Medical journals in developing countries

S NUNDY

Medical journals in developing countries are, with very few exceptions, unattractive. They contain poor science and are published late. In addition, they are rarely included in indexing services or referred to by researchers in either the developing or the developed worlds. Consequently, they constitute less than 5% of the world's cited scientific literature although developing countries have more than two thirds of the world's total population.

The causes for this sorry state of affairs are complex, and hard data on the subject are not available. In this analysis of Third World journals I will draw on the results of discussions with editorial colleagues in developing and developed countries; on the few publications on the subject; on my 10 years' experience of editing two medical journals in this region, *Tropical Gastroenterology* and *The National Medical Journal of India*; and on the results of a recently completed study on the quality of Indian medical journals, which we carried out for the Indian Council of Medical Research. I believe that this experience of Indian journals is fairly representative of medical journals in the rest of the Third World.

Reasons galore

The most important reason that Third World journals are of low quality is that there is a shortage of good medical research in these areas. Third World countries are poor, and governments tend to spend their scarce income on development projects and armaments rather than on health care and medical research. For instance, in 1989 India spent about one third of its budget on defence and only 1·9% on health care—a drop from the 4% that was allocated to health after independence 43 years ago. That this investment in medical research has yielded few worthwhile results has been emphasised in the speeches of the former Prime Minister, the late Rajiv Gandhi,[1] and this has discouraged the government from increasing research expenditure.

Universities and government centres are understaffed and technical personnel low paid and ill trained. The equipment available is outdated and much of it soon becomes non-functional because of inadequate maintenance services. Bureaucratic procedures handed down from the now distant colonial era cause delays not only in purchasing the most minor item of equipment but also in paying the suppliers. This deters foreign manufacturers from dealing with these countries.

The shortage of foreign currency and unfavourable exchange rates make it well nigh impossible for an individual doctor on an academic's salary to subscribe to any of the international journals. Most medical school libraries subscribe to only two or three journals and some to none at all. The foreign journals come by surface mail and arrive six months after their publication date, which enhances the feeling that we in the Third World are somewhat out of the mainstream. The best medical talent in these areas is drawn towards clinical practice because the financial rewards are much greater than in research and also because achievement in research carries with it much less prestige than does clinical competence. A large number of good papers does little to enhance an individual's prospects of advancement or promotion.

Although English is now the universal language of science, hostility to its use exists in many Indian states because it is identified with past foreign domination and is the language of the indigenous elite. English has been abolished as a medium of instruction in many primary schools and it has recently been banned by some states for interstate communication. Consequently, the standard of spoken and written English is deteriorating, and this is affecting the quality of Indian medical journals which use the language.

The best Indian researchers publish abroad because there is little prestige in having an article published in an Indian journal and because foreign journals have wider circulations, are better refereed, and are much more selective about accepting papers. For instance, in 1986, 66% of the 'most important' articles written by Fellows of the Indian National Science Academy were published in foreign journals—a generation ago only 23% were.[2] The articles rejected by foreign journals are offered to Indian journals. Here they are handled by part time staff who have little training in medical journalism. The articles are usually not acknowledged as having been received, are usually accepted without screening, and await their turn to be printed. A few journals send their articles to local referees, who may delay submitting their report for six months. Many referees consider the task to be more of a chore than an honour.

Once the material is gathered for publication little attention is paid to editing, proof reading, layout, and design. Then problems with production begin: paper is of poor quality; good printing presses are few; and even the best printers face many difficulties, including an intermittent supply of electricity. Production deadlines therefore remain unmet.

Doctors in the developing counrtries do not have a reading habit and the few that do (less than 5% in an informal survey)[3] read Western journals. The cause of this indifference to reading is a legacy of their experience in school and university, where learning is largely by rote and there is a consequent lack of interest in new ideas.

Quality and impact of Indian journals

In an interesting review of Indian science using citation data,[4] Garfield found that a wide range of subjects was covered but the quality of papers produced was poor. India ranked third in the world in scientific manpower (after the USA and the USSR) and eighth in the number of articles written (half the total Third World output), but the impact of the articles was very low. Articles in Indian journals were rarely cited by foreigners, and 90% of references in Indian articles were to foreign publications. Half the references were to articles more than 10 years old. These data, however, were derived from the few Indian journals included in the *Science Citation Index* and may therefore be providing an inaccurate perspective on Indian medical journal publishing.

Four years ago the Indian Council of Medical Research asked us to assess the quality of all Indian medical journals published in English. From a total of 382 Indian medical journals we excluded newsletters, drug company in house publications, homoeopathic and ayurvedic journals, and those that used languages other than English. We were left with 113 journals, which we analysed in some detail. They covered a wide range of subjects from anaesthesiology to urology and included genetics, parasitology, and social and preventive medicine (table), There were no weeklies, 19 month-

Subjects covered by Indian medical journals in 1985

Subject	No of journals covering subject
Anaesthesiology	3
Anatomy	1
Biochemistry	2
Cancer	2
Cardiovascular diseases	2
Chest diseases	2
Communicable diseases	2
Dermatology	3
Endocrinology	2
Ear, nose, and throat	2
Forensic medicine	1
Gastroenterology	2
General	33
General medicine	2
Genetics	2
Gerontology	1
Haematology	2
Hospital administration	1
Leprosy	1
Malariology	1
Microbiology	3
Neurology	2
Neuropsychiatry	2
Obstetrics and gynaecology	1
Ophthalmology	3
Orthopaedics	1
Paediatrics	5
Pathology	1
Parasitology	1
Pharmacology	2
Physiology	1
Plastic surgery	1
Psychiatry	5
Psychology	2
Radiology	2
Research	2
Rheumatology	1
Social and preventive medicine	5
Sports medicine	1
Surgery	2
Tuberculosis	2
Urology	1

lies, 11 bimonthlies, and 48 quarterlies. Most (90/113) were sponsored by professional societies and academic bodies and only four were brought out by private publishing firms. We assessed punctuality by the date a particular issue of a journal was received in the National Medical Library and found that only four journals came out on time in 1985 and the others were usually 1–12 months late. We sent the journals to Indian and foreign experts to assess their quality, and these experts felt that less than 20% were of international standards. The cumulated *Index Medicus* included 22, *Current Contents* three, and *Excerpta Medica* 26. A very disturbing revelation was the fact that most journals not included in the international indexing services did not deserve to be included and that Garfield had probably grossly overestimated the quality of Indian scientific journals.

Better medical writing

While this study was in progress a team from the *British Medical Journal* led by its editor, Stephen Lock, conducted a course entitled 'Better Medical Writing' at the All India Institute of Medical Sciences, New Delhi. The audience, from as far afield as Srinagar in the north of India and Trivandrum in the south, were enthused by this group of four Western editors and writers who discussed ways of improving the presentation of research results. There was lively discussion on conventional topics such as grammar, style, abstract length, and illustrations and on less conventional issues like: Are western editors prejudiced against articles from India? Should a paper published in a foreign journal carry more weight with a selection committee than one published in an Indian journal? and Does the quality of paper and typing influence an editor's choice? The proceedings were published as a small booklet (which has sold remarkably well).[5]

A new beginning

It was resolved at the end of this one day course that we should try to produce a first rate medical journal in India, and I was asked to be its editor. I invited eight others to form a working committee and we approached the government for financial support for this journal, to be called the *National Medical Journal of India*, which was readily agreed. From the *Index Medicus* for 1985 we made a list of the names and addresses of all authors with Indian sounding names— there were 355 in all in India and abroad—and wrote to them asking for contributions to our journal, offering a financial inducement of rupees 1000 (US$60) (not an insubstantial amount to an Indian academic) to authors whose articles we accepted.

To achieve Western standards we asked friends in Britain, USA, and India to help actively by becoming members of the editorial board, and we sent all articles to both Indian and foreign referees for assessment. We associated ourselves with a reputed publishing house, the Oxford University Press, and chose a printer who was deeply interested in his final product. We also computerised our production process to help us follow articles, choose and chase up referees, and pay authors by adapting a system that we had seen being used in London by the *British Medical Journal*. This reduced the number of errors entering the journal during its various stages of production. Our progress has been fairly encouraging. The number of papers received has gone up from 44 in the first four months of 1988 to 90 in the first four months of 1990, and our current rejection rate for original articles is 73%. We are now indexed in *Excerpta Medica*. We have at all stages sought help and advice from many friends in India and abroad, and this has been given unstintingly. They have all repeatedly stressed that we should not compromise on quality, however thin our issue turns out to be.

Other Third World editors might benefit by following our strategy, which consists essentially of first ensuring financial support for the journal for at least five years, asking for help from the most talented of their countrymen at home as well as those working in the West, being completely open to advice and criticism especially from experts, and using technology to minimise errors in production so as to speed up the publishing process and maintain quality. They should also get to know the best Western editors and unashamedly ask them for help because, as Garfield points out, we are part of an international community. Our experience has been that Western editors have been kind, considerate, yet unsparing in criticism; in short, their help has been invaluable.

How can Western editors help?

How can editors of established journals in the West help their colleagues in the developing countries? I think that they can do so as follows:

(1) By offering continuous background support. This is needed in many different ways including helping with refereeing, checking references, suggesting potential authors, and providing feedback on the final product. There is a genuine fear among Third World editors that all this might incite a patronising attitude, but when there is such a difference in standards it should matter little what attitude is adopted.

79

(2) By training editorial staff. This can be done by very short courses of the 'travelling circus' type or by providing fellowships to editors from developing countries to work in the offices of established journals for short periods of up to six months. Experience with technological innovations may lead to their adapting some of these to their own home situations.

(3) By giving 'how to' books on editing, old issues of Western journals, and outmoded technology (such as discarded personal computers) to the Third World editors. The books and journals can be used to build up a reference library that will be accessible to the production staff as showing standards of quality. The technology that is out of date in say, Britain, may be most appropriate for India's present stage of development.

Finally, until the quality of Third World journals improves substantially, Western editors can help Third World medical research further as follows:

(1) By treating papers submitted by authors in developing countries 'sympathetically,' realising that the quality of typing may be substandard but the science may be interesting and good, and when a paper is rejected by sending a detailed report to the authors pointing out its weaknesses and suggesting how the work might be improved.

(2) By including in Western journals articles that might be useful to Third World doctors. The medical leaders in developing countries still read mainly Western journals and will continue to be influenced by them for the forseeable future.

A sustained effort over several years might help to improve the quality of medical journals in developing countries and it might also assist our search for answers to some of the Third World's medical problems. It will certainly forge new and warm personal friendships.

1 Gandhi R. Indian science must be equal to the best. Address to the concluding session of the 73rd Indian Science Congress. New Delhi, 7 January 1986. Reported in: Express News Service. PM for management concept in science. *Indian Express* 1986 Jan 8;1(cols 2–4).
2 Krishnan CN, Visvanathan B. The performance of modern science and technology in India: the case of scientific and technological journals. *Patriotic and People Oriented Science and Technology Bulletin* 1987;11:1–19.
3 Bose S, Nundy S. Indian medical journals—a critical review. *Trop Gastroenterol* 1984;5:107–11.
4 Garfield E. Third World research. Part I. Where it is published and how often it is cited. *Current Contents* 1983;33:6–15.
5 Lock S, Smith J, Whimster W. Paton A. *Better medical writing in India.* New Delhi: The National Medical Journal of India, 1986.

Mapping the land of medical journals: some new applications for citation data from *Science Citation Index*

EDWARD J HUTH

Journals in medicine are not a homogeneous set of publications. They often differ greatly in scope, in quality, in audience, and in utility. Being able to distinguish among them is valuable to many persons affected in one way or another by medical information, its availability, and its flow: authors, readers, editors, and librarians. Judging journals' characteristics and values is easy enough for persons who know well the journals they seek to judge and know what their content represents. Persons not so equipped may be able to accept judgements from colleagues that may represent both individual judgements and widely perceived reputations of the journals. But a reputation can run on long after change in a journal's character and value. And there are journals not well known or known at all by available and reliable colleagues.

Judgements of these kinds are usually subjective, impressionistic. They rarely can give a clear picture of how journals relate to each other and where they stand in the stream of medical information as it flows from its origins in basic science to the clinician. Objective and quantitative methods for assessing journals' qualities and how journals relate to each other may offer more reliable and consistent judgements and a more detailed picture than those derived from subjective, impressionistic, ad hoc judgements.

81

More precise estimates of influence and hierarchy

Bibliometric methods for analysing and describing how information is generated, distributed, and judged already are the basis for many published reports about information science.[1] Quantitative methods in citation analysis have been used for several decades to assess journals' influence and positions. The best known of these methods are those developed by Eugene Garfield[2][3] and Henry Small: the calculations based on the citation data in the *Science Citation Index* (*SCI*) database of the Institute for Scientific Information and reported annually in the *Journal Citation Reports* volume of the *SCI*. These calculations yield the *SCI* 'impact factor' and 'immediacy index', explained in the introduction to *Journal Citation Reports*[4] and presented in various formats in the *Reports*.

If journals are ranked in importance simply by the degree to which their papers are cited (the total number of citations in a given year) those journals publishing many papers are likely to have their papers cited more often than those publishing few papers. The impact factor adjusts for this potential bias in ranking by dividing the number of citations of a journal's papers by the number of citable papers ('source items') that the journal published in a given period. The premise behind this calculation assumes that all papers are of equal merit and hence equally likely to be cited. If the citation rate is adjusted for the number of papers a journal publishes, therefore, the resulting impact factor reflects the average importance or influence of its papers. Specifically, the impact factor represents the number of citations (by the papers in all of the journals represented in the *SCI* database) of a journal's papers in a given year divided by the number of the journal's source items published in the preceding two years. The formula is:

$$\text{Impact factor} = \frac{\text{Citations of a journal's papers in all } SCI \text{ journals}}{\text{Papers it published in the preceding two years}}$$

Thus the impact factor represents a journal by an average number of citations per paper published.

The other assessment factor reported annually in *Journal Citation Reports* is the immediacy index, a measure of how quickly a journal's papers are cited after their publication. This index does not enter the considerations of this chapter and will not be discussed further.

The data and methods in this chapter

The data used for the calculations represented in this chapter have been drawn from the citation data and indices reported in the *Journal Citation Reports* volume of the 1988 *Science Citation Index*.[4] The formulas are explained in the three following sections and their premises defined. Possible reservations about what the factors produced by the formulas represent are set forth.

The scope adjusted impact factor: a refinement of the 'impact factor'

As explained above, the impact factor reflects the degree to which a journal's papers are cited in all journals represented in the *SCI* database, adjusted for the number of papers the journal pubishes. The calculation does not make any adjustment for the scope of the journal, which does appear to be a determinant of the probability that its papers will be cited. If a journal publishes only papers representing a small discipline its papers will probably influence the content of only a few journals; hence the annual numbers of citations of its papers should be relatively small. If a journal publishes papers representing a wide range of topics through many disciplines, its papers are likely to be cited in many journals, which will probably result in a relatively large number of citations. Hence it seems reasonable to adjust further the number of citations of a journal's papers (as represented within the impact factor) for the scope of the journal. The figure shows the general correlation between the scope of a journal as represented by the number of journals citing its papers and the average number of citations its papers receive (the impact factor) in the entire *SCI* group of journals (although there are some conspicuous outliers from this correlation). The impact factor does not take into account the topical scope of journals; its calculation assumes that all papers published by the journals represented in the *SCI* database are of equal potential importance to all authors publishing in all of these journals.

The calculation of the scope adjusted impact factor (SA impact factor) adjusts the impact factor for the scope of journals by dividing a journal's impact factor by the number of journals citing its papers. This datum is available in the Cited Journal Listing section of *Journal Citations Reports*.[4] It must be noted here, for a reason discussed below, that this number appears to be the total number of journals that have cited a journal's papers through all the years for

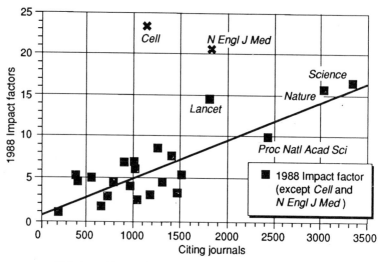

FIGURE —*Relation of impact factor to number of citing journals (as measure of scope). Because Cell and the New England Journal of Medicine appeared to be outliers, their data were excluded from the calculation of the linear regression line.*

which citation data for it have appeared in the *SCI*, and not just the number of journals citing its papers in the two immediately preceding years that determine the impact factor. The basic formula for this calculation is:

$$\text{Scope adjusted impact factor} = \frac{\text{Impact factor}}{\text{Number of citing journals}}$$

The division by the large numbers in the denominators produces numbers that are smaller than the impact factors by a factor of around 1000. To bring the SA impact factor back to a magnitude akin to that of the impact factor, the calculation multiplies the resulting decimal fraction by 1000. Hence the formula for the SA impact factor becomes:

$$\text{Scope adjusted impact factor} = \frac{\text{Impact factor}}{\text{Number of citing journals}} \times 1000$$

SA impact factors have been calculated for 25 journals that represent a cluster of journals important in clinical medicine or whose data illustrate the new insights yielded by this calculation.

84

TABLE I — *Scope adjusted (SA) impact factors (ImpFs) with journal rankings by this factor*

	1988 ImpF	Rank by ImpF (in this group)	No of citing journals (CJ)	SA impact factor (ImpF/ CJ) ×1000
Cell	23·91	1	1127	21·22
J Am Coll Cardiol	5·20	13	383	13·58
N Engl J Med	21·15	2	1819	11·63
J Clin Oncol	4·60	15	411	11·19
Hepatology	4·95	14	552	8·97
Lancet	14·48	5	1788	8·10
Circulation	6·68	10	896	7·46
Blood	6·85	9	1003	6·83
Ann Intern Med	8·47	7	1253	6·76
Gastroenterology	6·13	11	1019	6·02
Am J Psychiatry	4·31	17	786	5·48
J Clin Invest	7·59	8	1408	5·39
Nature	15·76	4	3002	5·25
Science	16·46	3	3320	4·96
Am Rev Respir Dis	4·48	16	961	4·66
J Clin Endocrinol Metab	4·09	19	976	4·19
Proc Natl Acad Sci USA	10·03	6	2418	4·15
Am J Cardiol	2·62	22	720	3·64
JAMA	5·28	12	1515	3·49
Cancer Res	4·30	18	1305	3·30
Am J Hosp Pharm	0·65	25	220	2·96
Chest	1·59	24	658	2·42
Am J Med	2·73	21	1180	2·31
Cancer	2·24	23	1042	2·15
BMJ	3·14	20	1469	2·14

Table I gives the data applied in, and coming from, the calculation; it shows the advantage of the SA impact factor over the impact factor for more accurate assessment of a journal's influence *within its topical scope* (italics added for emphasis). The journals are ranked by their SA impact factors, but their rankings by impact factor are also represented. Several effects of the calculation are represented by some changes in ranking. The broad scope journals *Nature, Proceedings of the National Academy of Sciences*, and *Science* rank high by the impact factor (4, 6 and 3, respectively among the 25 journals analysed). Ranked by the SA impact factor, they rank 13, 17, and 14, respectively. We may judge that, although their 'impact' is substantial within the entire scope of journals represented in the *SCI*, their 'impact' on specific fields within this entire scope is relatively less than that of the journals in those specific fields. The reverse effect is seen for relatively narrow scope journals, virtually all of which move up in ranking, several quite strikingly. The narrow scope journals *Hepatology* and *Journal of Clinical Oncology*, ranked 14 and 15 by the impact factor, move up to ranks 5 and 4 for the SA impact factor. Thus these two journals appear to be highly influential within their fields.

It must be noted, however, that both of them were founded relatively recently and hence the number of journals whose papers have cited them may be relatively low compared with those for journals that have been published for many more years. Papers in a journal that has been published for many years may be cited occasionally in journals relatively peripheral to its main field, and these citations would tend to suggest a wider scope for a journal than is accurate. Note, for example, that the *Journal of the American College of Cardiology*, founded quite recently, ranks conspicuously higher than *Circulation*, which has been published for many more years. Is this difference in rank due mainly to the effect of length of time in which citations, and hence the numbers of citing journals, can have accumulated? Or does it represent a real difference, article by article, in influence? There may be methods available for adjusting the SA impact factor for the possible effect of duration of publication, but I have not explored the possibilities enough to discuss them here.

Possible use of rankings of journals by apparent scope as judged by numbers of citing journals

If the number of journals that cite the papers of a particular journal is a reasonable measure of its scope (the size and number of the disciplines it represents) this number could be used in judgments by librarians and potential subscribers in selecting journals for their scope as general journals or specialised journals. Table II ranks the 25 journals sampled for this analysis by the number of journals citing their papers. Such a ranking could be applied, for example, to selecting journals for 'core libraries' by taking the most influential journal (for a field particularly important for the library), as identified by the influence factor, and then identifying the titles of the journals that the journal most influences; this information can come from an analysis of journal specific factors, the subject of the next section.

The journal specific influence factor

Both the *SCI* impact factor and the scope adjusted impact factor serve only as indexes of the influence papers published in a journal

TABLE II — *Scope of journals reflected by numbers of citing journals*

	1988 ImpF	Rank by ImpF	No of citing journals (CJ)	SA impact factor (ImpF/CJ) ×1000	Rank by SA impact factor
Science	16·46	3	3320	4·96	14
Nature	15·76	4	3002	5·25	13
Proc Natl Acad Sci USA	10·03	6	2418	4·15	17
New Engl J Med	21·15	2	1819	11·63	3
Lancet	14·48	5	1788	8·10	6
JAMA	5·28	12	1515	3·49	19
BMJ	3·14	20	1469	2·14	25
J Clin Invest	7·59	8	1408	5·39	12
Cancer Res	4·30	18	1305	3·30	20
Ann Intern Med	8·47	7	1253	6·76	9
Am J Med	2·73	21	1180	2·31	23
Cell	23·91	1	1127	21·22	1
Cancer	2·24	23	1042	2·15	24
Gastroenterology	6·13	11	1019	6·02	10
Blood	6·85	9	1003	6·83	8
J Clin Endocrinol Metab	4·09	19	976	4·19	16
Am Rev Respir Dis	4·48	16	961	4·66	15
Circulation	6·68	10	896	7·46	7
Am J Psychiatry	4·31	17	786	5·48	11
Am J Cardiol	2·62	22	720	3·64	18
Chess	1·59	24	658	2·42	22
Hepatology	4·95	14	552	8·97	5
J Clin Oncol	4·60	15	411	11·19	4
J Am Coll Cardiol	5·20	13	383	13·58	2
Am J Hosp Pharm	0·65	25	220	2·96	21

ImpF = impact factor

have on the other papers published in a set of journals. The impact factor probably overestimates a broad scope journal's influence and underestimates the influence of a narrow scope journal within its specific field. The scope adjusted impact factor probably more accurately estimates a journal's influence within the discipline (or disciplines) it represents. Neither factor indicates a journal's influence on the papers in other individual journals (or those in itself). For a measure of the influence of the papers in one journal on those in another, I propose the journal specific influence factor.

Calculation of this factor for a specific journal is based on the numbers of citations of its papers in the papers in the 'influenced' journals being considered, with adjustments for the number of source items (original articles, reviews) in the journal cited and the number of source items in the 'influenced' journal. These adjustments are based on the premises that the more source items a journal publishes the more likely that its papers will be cited and that the more source items (papers) the 'influenced' journal publishes the more citations it will carry. These adjustments are akin to that applied for the *SCI* impact factor, in the calculation of which the number of citations to a journal's papers is divided by the number of the source items it publishes so that the factor measures the average citation rate of its individual papers. The divisors that make these adjustments are applied in the formula as square roots so that the product denominator in the formula is of the same general magnitude as the numbers of source items for individual journals. (It should be noted that this pair of square root factors produces in the formula applied to estimating the influence of a journal's papers on itself a divisor that is the number of source items in the journal.) Thus the formula for calculating the journal specific influence factor (JSIF) representing the influence of journal A (Jrl A) on journal B (Jrl B) is as follows:

$$\text{JSIF for A on B} = \frac{\text{Citations in Jrl B of Jrl A's source items}}{\sqrt{(\text{Jrl A SIs})} \times \sqrt{(\text{Jrl B SIs})}} \times 1000$$

where SIs are the number of source items. In the calculation the number of citations is for one year (in this paper, 1988) and the source item numbers are the average of source items for 1987 and 1986.

Tables III and IV show the journal specific influence factors thus calculated for the *New England Journal of Medicine* and the *Annals of Internal Medicine*. The data are given for only the top 25 citing journals as ranked by the factor (although factors were calculated for 75 journals). The first columns give the ranking of the citing journals by the total numbers of citations in 1988 to the 1986 and 1987 papers published in the two journals considered. The total numbers of citations of articles in these two journals appear to be influenced by the scope and numbers of source items published by the respective journals, but also by the relation of the scope of a journal to that of the cited journal. The effect of the calculation in allowing for the 'size' (number of citing source items) of a journal is strikingly seen in the influence factors of the two journals for *AIDS*, a journal publishing a relatively small number of papers; in relation to both cited journals, *AIDS* moved up in rank quite sharply. The *New England Journal of Medicine* 'influenced' *AIDS* as heavily as it 'influenced' the other relatively wide scope journals (*JAMA*, *Lancet*, and *Annals of Internal Medicine*) ; this heavy influence could not

TABLE III — *The New England Journal of Medicine: its journal specific influence factors (JSIFs) for 25 journals, compared with ranking by NEJM citations* in those journals*

Journals ranked by 1988 citations*	1988 Citations* of NEJM papers	Journals ranked by JSFs	JIFs
N Engl J Med	2154	N Engl J Med	2·08
JAMA	1017	AIDS	0·86
Lancet	987	JAMA	0·83
Am J Med	856	Lancet	0·82
Ann Intern Med	819	Ann Intern Med	0·81
Am J Cardiol	805	J Am Coll Cardiol	0·55
J Am Coll Cardiol	683	Dis J Infect	0·41
Am Heart J	606	Am J Cardiol	0·40
Blood	584	Am J Med	0·40
Arch Intern Med	554	Internist (Berlin)	0·36
BMJ	520	Arch Intern Med	0·36
J Infect Dis	503	Blood	0·35
Chest	492	Am Heart J	0·34
Cancer	490	Clin Perinatol	0·33
Am Rev Respir Dis	484	Dtsch Med Wochesnschr	0·33
Transpl Proc	476	Pediatr Clin North Am	0·32
Circulation	441	BMJ	0·32
Cancer Res	435	Schweiz Med Wochenschr	0·30
Dtsch Med Wochenschr	422	Circulation	0·30
J Pediatr	418	Med Clin North Am	0·30
J Clin Invest	385	Presse Med	0·29
Transplantation	338	Am J Public Health	0·29
Med Clin North Am	333	Mayo Clin Proc	0·27
Schweiz Med Wochenschr	326	Pediatr Infect Dis	0·27
Pediatr Infect Dis	310	Z Kardiol	0·26

* 1988 Citations of articles in *New England Journal of Medicine* in 1986 and 1987

have been guessed simply from the total number of citations in *AIDS* of papers published in the *New England Journal*. In general, the rankings by influence of the cited journals of relatively narrow-scope journals that publish large numbers of papers, such as *Blood*, *American Review of Respiratory Disease*, and *Cancer Research* drop. With regard to the *Annals*, it is striking that among the journals most heavily 'influenced' are synoptic journals like *Gastroenterology Clinics of North America*, *Disease of the Month*, and *Seminars in Hematology*. These journals' citations would have to be examined in an attempt to uncover the basis for these rankings; my speculation is that the basis may lie in the *Annals* having put considerable emphasis on publishing reviews (formal reviews, conferences, and so on) that themselves serve as substantial synoptic sources. The

TABLE IV — *Annals of Internal Medicine: its journal specific influence factors (JSIFs) for 25 journals, compared with ranking by Annals citations* in those journals*

Journals ranked by 1988 citations*	1988 Citations* of Annals papers	Journals ranked by JSIFs	JSIFs
Ann Intern Med	315	*Ann Intern Med*	1·17
Am J Med	137	*AIDS*	0·89
JAMA	115	*Gastroenterol Clin North Am*	0·57
N Engl J Med	108	*Clin Chest Med*	0·41
AIDS	91	*Dis Mon*	0·39
Arch Intern Med	78	*Semin Hematol*	0·37
Chest	63	*N Engl J Med*	0·35
J Infect Dis	62	*Am J Med*	0·32
Am J Cardiol	62	*JAMA*	0·30
Lancet	61	*Arch Intern Med*	0·26
Gastroenterol Clin North Am	49	*Med Clin North Am*	0·21
Clin Chest Med	49	*Medicine (Baltimore)*	0·21
BMJ	45	*J Infect Dis*	0·21
Am J Gastroenterol	44	*Mayo Clin Proc*	0·19
Dtsch Med Wochenschr	44	*Am J Gastroenterol*	0·17
Press Med	42	*Chest*	0·17
Schweiz Med Wochenschr	40	*Lancet*	0·17
J Am Coll Cardiol	39	*Am J Med Sci*	0·17
Am Rev Respir Dis	38	*Presse Med*	0·16
Semin Hematol	35	*Rheum Dis Clin North Am*	0·15
Blood	35	*Rev Infect Dis*	0·15
Mayo Clin Proc	34	*Drug Intell Clin Pharm*	0·15
Rev Infect Disect	34	*Dtsch Med Wochenschr*	0·14
J Clin Oncol	34	*Schweitz Med Wochenschr*	0·14
West J Med	34	*J Clin Oncol*	0·14

* 1988 Citations articles in *Annals of Internal Medicine* in 1986 and 1987

Annals has also tended to publish descriptive articles (in contrast to bench research, trials, and epidemiological reports) as a larger fraction of its contents than have journals such as the *New England Journal*.

Maps of information flow

Obviously the journal specific influence factors can be used to assess how the papers in a particular journal influence the content of other journals, as that influence can be estimated from citations. Another use I intend to explore is the development of 'maps' of the flow of information among journals. If one calculates the JSIF for two journals as cited journal and citing journal pairs, those factors suggest the net balance of influence on each other. For example, the *New England Journal's* JSIF for the *Annals* is 0·81; that of the *Annals* for the *New England Journal* is 0·35. The net flow can be judged as being from the *New England Journal* to the *Annals*. An adjustment for degree of specialisation of the two journals would probably have to be applied; relatively narrow scope journals like *Blood* and *Circulation* would not be expected to influence heavily the total content of the *New England Journal*.

Developing such maps will take far more time than is available for preparing this chapter, but I hope eventually to report and display the results after I have had enough time to think through the conceptual basis for such maps and an effective means of representing them graphically.

Limits of interpretation

Care must be taken in interpreting citation data. The limits of their usefulness have been pointed out by Garfield[5] and others, but some merit brief discussion here. Some of these limits are well known to all who have given any thought to possible applications of citation data. Methods papers tend to get cited heavily, and especially influential methods papers tend to be cited much more than reports of even highly influential research.[6] This aspect of citation data generally is of little importance in judging clinical journals' influence; clinical journals may contribute heavily to citations of methods papers in basic science and laboratory science journals, but themselves rarely publish methods papers. Attention has also been drawn to the citing of papers in 'negative' judgements of their contents; this phenomenon must be considered to be an influence even though it could be described as a pejorative kind of influence.

Special care should be taken in applying citation data to judgements of how journals influence clinical practice in contrast to continuing research. Citation data drawn from primary journals probably tend to reflect conceptual, rather than practical, influence, at least to the extent that the cited papers are research reports rather than synoptic papers. The translation of research results to changes in practice probably depends heavily on the processing of primary papers by writers of review articles and textbooks and by teachers in medical schools and postgraduate programmes. One approach to assessing journals' probable practical influence has considered whether textbook citations are a more reliable basis for identifying the most influential sources of information with clear clinical relevance.[7]

Possible uses of these bibliometric measures and conclusion

The *SCI* impact factor has long seemed to me to be a crude, not notably discriminating approach to judging the influence of journals on each other and their direct influence on the practice of medicine. There is ample evidence that journals are substantially more important to investigators and clinical academicians than to practising doctors. Editors who see themselves as hoping to influence practice desirably and effectively need objective means of judging what they do, how they do it, and its consequences. Two other groups of possible users of more refined methods for analysing citation data are librarians and abstracters. Some of the methods described here could be applied to defining more accurately 'core libraries' and to selecting journals for surveillance by abstracters and writers of synoptic papers.

In this chapter I have suggested some quantitative methods for coming to clearer insights into the effects and values of journals. The calculations suggested have not, obviously, had any external validation, but I have indicated the premises on which they are based so that the reasonableness of these approaches can at least be discussed and tested further.

1 Borgman CL, ed. *Scholarly communication and bibliometrics*. Newbury Park, California: Sage Publications, 1990.
2 Garfield E. Citation analysis as a tool in journal evaluation. *Science* 1972;**178**:471–9.
3 Garfield E. *Citation indexing: its theory and application in science, technology, and humanities*. New York: John Wiley, 1979.
4 Garfield E, ed. *Journal citation reports. Science citation index*, vol 19. Philadelphia: Institute for Science Information, 1988.
5 Garfield E. Uses and misuses of citation frequency. *Current Contents (Life Sciences)* 1985;**28**(No 43)(Oct 28):3–9.
6 Garfield E. The most-cited papers of all time, *SCI* 1945–1988: Part 1A. The top 100—will the Lowry method ever be obliterated? *Current Contents* 1990;**33**(Feb 12):3–14.
7 Zlotogorski A, Israeli A. The use of textbooks in evaluating the impact of medical journals. *Can Med Assoc J* 1988;**138**:685–6.

Research agenda for medical journals

SUZANNE W FLETCHER

This chapter starts with the proposition that medical journals can, and indeed should, undertake investigative activities into the editorial process.[1] To my knowledge, no medical journal engages in ongoing research into its editorial processes; most do not even undertake occasional studies. It is a bit ironic that there is not yet a strong tradition among medical journals to study their activities. Editors generally come from a research background, and journals publishing original research participate in an effort that at its heart demands that those who think they know something subject their ideas to scientific scrutiny. So, on philosophical grounds alone, one might make the argument that scientific investigation of ourselves and our craft is a good idea.

Most medical editors would agree that scientific inquiry is not only important but stimulating as well. Perhaps editing would be more fun if we preserved a little time to continue the practice of science as well as to read about it. It is even possible that continuing to practise research will make us better readers and editors of science.

The current social climate also argues for investigation of the editorial process. Medical journals no longer merely speak to the few academic physicians who might be inclined to read them, as was probably true 50 years ago. Today, the articles published in medical journals receive extensive lay press coverage. This is especially true in North America for large medical journals such as the *New England Journal of Medicine* and the *Journal of the American Medical Association*, but it is also true for many others. For instance, issues of *Annals of Internal Medicine* go not only to 95 000 medical subscribers but also to over 300 newspapers, news bureaux, and television and radio stations. In May and June of 1990, articles in the *Annals* were cited more than 1300 times in the lay media. Although I do not know the comparable figures, certainly the numbers are even larger for the *New England Journal of Medicine* and the *Journal of the American Medical Association.*

Because medical journals now speak to society as well, their impact can be more profound. In April 1990 the *Annals* published an article that suggested an association between a non-steroidal anti-inflammatory drug and renal failure. In the weeks after publication of that article, over 700 newspapers in the United States covered the study, almost certainly because of public concern about an extensively used medication.

Other recent events point to the growing influence of medical journals, at least in the United States. Concerns about whether the peer review process itself is delaying vital medical information getting to physicians and patients indicate the importance critics assign to the process. Such critics clearly do not think the activities in medical editorial offices are ivory tower irrelevancies. The growing governmental concern about fraud in medical reseach also affects medical journals. In such an environment, medical journals need to adopt the best possible processes to ensure the best possible publications in our journals, and to scrutinise ourselves and our activities in the best scientific tradition.

A proposed framework for investigations

Many different frameworks could be used for research on medical editing. One useful framework, however, comes from clinical epidemiological research. Basic to that discipline are clinical questions about defining and diagnosing disease or medical conditions, assessing incidences, searching for risk factors and deciding their relative importance, clarifying clinical course and prognosis, and evaluating treatment and preventive strategies. These questions are studied with epidemiological methods of cross sectional studies and surveys, prospective studies, case control investigations, and clinical trials, usually culminating with randomised controlled trials. Depending on the question asked, one or another method is most appropriate for the study.

How can medical editors who want to investigate what they are doing make use of such an approach? Research presented at the First International Congress on Peer Review in Biomedical Publication can be used as illustration. Investigations into who, what, and how much peer reviewers do[2][3]; the editorial processes of different journals[4] [5]; and quotational and reference accuracy in surgical journals[6] were cross sectional studies determining frequencies and definitions. A cohort study of summary reports of controlled trials investigated the natural course of such trials.[7] 'Treatments' such as statistical assessment of papers[8] and blinding of reviewers[9] were evaluated with an uncontrolled trial and a randomised controlled trial.

Some suggestions for a research agenda

Ideas for research in medical editing probably should evolve in much the same manner as they do for clinical research, beginning with an experience that raises questions and stimulates investigation, which in turn leads to further research. Partly because I have been involved in only two investigations of editing, most of my ideas come from the first part of the chain of events, rather than from previous research. (There has been remarkably little research overall in medical editing, certainly not yet enough to support a 'Journal of Medical Editing Research'.)

In our first jobs as editors, for the *Journal of General Internal Medicine*, Robert Fletcher and I became fascinated by the complexity of the peer review process for our journal. We found ourselves trying to define a 'good review'. By attempting to study how to improve peer review, we were forced to come up with an operational definition of a 'good review'. We barely scratched the investigative surface in this endeavour. To define 'good review' in a scientifically rigorous and editorially useful way, the definition that is developed should be subjected to and should pass the usual tests of validity and reliability that scientists require of all important definitions in research.

Perhaps more rewarding would be intervention research to evaluate strategies to improve peer review. (Of course, it is very hard to study possible improvements if the entity cannot be defined in the first place. Thus, the need for work on definitions.) With colleagues at the University of North Carolina we evaluated the effect on the quality of the reviewers' work of blinding reviewers to the identity of authors.[9] We found that, by our definition, the quality of the reviews improved with blinding. What about evaluating other interventions, such as identifying the reviewers, paying them, or publicly acknowledging them? In answer to modern critics, why not study carefully whether and what peer review adds to the editorial selection process and the quality of published articles?

Another general topic needing investigation is the relation between medical journals and authors of submitted manuscripts. Over the past several years editors have indicated increasing concern about duplicate or repetitive publication and 'salami science'. If the problem of duplicate publication were to be studied according to the clinical epidemiological framework I have outlined, some of the following questions might be tackled. First, diagnostic studies are needed. Do editors, authors, and reviewers diagnose, or define, duplicate publishing in the same way? What is the incidence of the phenomenon? What are the risk factors for duplicate publishing? What is the natural history of such authors; are there chronic offenders, or is the problem sporadic? Finally, what is the effect of various interventions?

A similar approach could be used to study the quality of accepted manuscripts and how to improve their scientific content[8] and their format.

Some might say that the agenda set out above is impossible, too much is unknown, medical editing is too much an art based on experience, and editors have too little time for medical journals to be fertile soil for scientific investigations. I am sure that editors, who, more than most, know the value of the scientific method to study questions and ideas, will disagree. In fact, for science to contribute to medical editing, it must be editors who promote and engage in the studies.

Suggestions on how to conduct research on medical editing

Because the research agenda for medical editing is large, and because it takes a great deal of time and effort to tackle even a single research question, progress might be made much more quickly if editors worked together. Dr Drummond Rennie began a cooperative venture of editors into medical editing research when he organised the research symposium on peer review. He is now organising the second congress. This is a wonderful initiative, but further progress is needed. Obviously, such endeavors should continue. But why not add to them by beginning collaborative research efforts? In exactly that spirit, the National Library of Medicine has funded the preliminary discussions of several medical journals to undertake a collaborative evaluation of blinding in peer review. I hope this beginning effort will develop successfully, not only for the project at hand, but for continuing collaborative research in medical editing.

Collaborative research work among medical journals will not be easy, not only because of logistical problems, but also because funding will have to be obtained. The natural competitiveness among journals might also make collaboration difficult. But gains for the discipline of medical editing might be substantial.

I have attempted to lay out some reasons for developing investigative activities in medical editing, suggested one framework for such investigations, given a few examples of topics that might make up a research agenda, and finally suggested that editors develop ways to pursue research both individually and collectively. Having entered the medical editing world on a full time basis only very recently, I am still impressed at what a small group it is that has such awesome responsibility for so much. To do our very best to meet the responsibility of modern medical editing, we must use the best art and science we can muster.

1 Bailar JC, Patterson K. Journal peer review: the need for a research agenda. *N Engl J Med* 1985;**312**:654–7.
2 Yankauer A, Who are the peer reviewers and how much do they review? *JAMA* 1990;**263**:1338–40.
3 Lock S, Smith J. What do peer reviewers do? *JAMA* 1990;**263**:1341–3.
4 Weller A. Editorial peer review in US medical journals. *JAMA* 1990;**263**:1344–7.
5 Hargens L. Variation in journal peer review systems. Possible causes and consequences. *JAMA* 1990;**263**:1348–52.
6 Evans JT, Nadjari HI, Burchell, SA. Quotational and reference accuracy in surgical journals. A continuing peer review problem. *JAMA* 1990;**263**:1353–4.
7 Chalmers I, Adams M, Dickersin K, *et al.* A cohort study of summary reports of controlled trials. *JAMA* 1990:**263**:1401–5.
8 Gardner MJ, Bond J. An exploratory study of statistical assessment of papers published in the British Medical Journal. *JAMA* 1990:**263**:1355–7.
9 McNutt RA, Evans AT, Fletcher RH, Fletcher, SW. The effects of blinding on the quality of peer review. A randomized trial. *JAMA* 1990;**263**:1371–6.

PART 3
THE COMMUNICATION OF CLINICAL INFORMATION

The changing editorial paradigm: hard data are necessary but no longer sufficient conditions for publishing clinical trials

POVL RIIS

The process of editing scientific journals has changed radically during the past 50 years. Fifty years ago editors were mostly appointed for what they were, and not what they could be, having learned what later appeared to be a specialty in itself. Editorial policies then reflected an era before the advent of randomised controlled trials; the clinical medicine community knew no better and failed to consider its own concepts and methods critically. Its members went on in the traditional way without realising that a paradigm shift was rapidly approaching.

The era before randomised controlled trials

The history of medicine is full of fallacious conclusions about the effects of treatment. Leaving the magic methods and demonic interpretations to remain in prehistoric darkness—an exclusion probably too fair to contemporary, global medicine—enables us to concentrate on the lifetime of the oldest western European and North Atlantic general medical journals. During most of this time the influence of the 'Geheimrat' system declined gradually, and the legions of anecdotal reports gradually became replaced by those characterised by numerical methods. Counting and calculating became acknowledged techniques, but were still without the necessary apparatus of the sources of the figures which would have enabled the scientist and the reader to go behind the figures and ask: How were they gathered? How representative are they? How strong is their predictive force?

The prodromal signs of a paradigm shift came from outside, in the first place from the statisticians. Names such as 'Student',[1] Pearson,[2] Fisher,[3] Bradford-Hill,[4] Witts,[5] Mainland,[6] and many others gradually opened the eyes of clinical scientists and editors. This final stage of the era before randomised controlled trials lasted at most half a century, because of the traditional master and apprenticeship principle of medical education and the slowness with which scientific concepts and designs were applied in clinical medicine. To teach scientists, readers, and editors, that 'all judgements rest on comparisons' and that 'everything varies' in human biology took time, because a middle aged clinician's acceptance of these theses was considered to be a personal verdict—'Not capable of thinking stringently until today.' But slowly the theses indicated the necessity of a new paradigm in clinical research. When comparisons became necessary for all scientific judgements, evaluating therapeutic effects made the introduction of control groups necessary; unbiased judgements similarly made it necessary to control psychological bias by blinding; and the ever varying nature of human biology and disease states demanded that variation should be distributed evenly by randomisation. Furthermore, to distinguish such stochastic distributions from variations caused by intervention it became necessary to apply numerical calculations of random distribution—the so called significance tests. During the late 1940s and the 1950s these principles became adopted by the high priests of medicine, and the era of the randomised controlled trial was proclaimed.

The era of randomised controlled trials

Editors became part of the new developments. They even had to be trained themselves to apply the new methods—how to plan, carry through, and interpret clinical research projects. They *had* to, realising that you cannot lead an organisation if you do not understand it, while still avoiding the other extreme—that to know too many details is to get bogged down in tactics and forget to be a strategist. Authors realised that a new era had arrived, because titles such as 'Seventeen depressed patients treated with a new antidepressant' were now repeatedly rejected with laconic messages; 'Sorry, no room for uncontrolled therapeutic studies'.

As in the case of other powerful new movements, the era of the randomised controlled trial sometimes made scientists and editors 'more royalist than the king'. Statistical methods and their cabalistic symbols swarmed over journal pages like contagious agents. Even weak studies became impressive (to the extent of deceiving editors) if sufficient p values were scattered throughout the manuscript. Significance tests were applied, sometimes in a way that disclosed the inability of authors, reviewers, editors, and readers to see the false goddesses of the p value. Investigators, for instance, grouped their obese patients into subgroups with moderate and severe adiposity, calculated means for the body weights of both groups, and triumphantly stated that the intergroup difference was significant. Or authors calculated the mean age of a large group of patients and compared it with the mean age of the same group at follow up two years later. Again the message to innocent readers was the revolutionary one that two years make people older.

The adoration of the p even led some scientists to apply, and editors to demand, the principles of the controlled trial when they were not needed. Other problems arose—for instance, using randomised controlled trials in rare diseases which necessitated multicentre trials, with new demands for controlling bias not only within a group but also among separate groups.

After the initial wave of religious awe towards biostatistics (often much regretted by the statisticians), a second development of understanding has slowly appeared. Such understanding has become manifest in the interest in clinical definitions, the existence of type II errors (a true intergroup difference being masked by non-systematic variation within small groups), the concept of MIREDIF (the minimal relevant difference to be sought for in clinical trials), research ethics, etc.

At the end of the era of the randomised controlled trial we can now detect the enormous positive impact it has had on clinical science and publication. This positive influence is shown particularly in the modifications introduced in the interactions between statistics and clinical science, now reflected in editorial policies.

One major step forward, for instance, has been the increasing use of confidence intervals instead of p values over, or below, that magic borderline of 0·01 or 0·05. Instead of presenting readers with a kind of command on how to interpret results, authors now accept readers as equals and let them judge for themselves through confidence intervals.

The era after randomised controlled trials

The approaching era after the randomised controlled trial will not entail a radical shift of the editorial paradigm: an-out-with-that-in-with-this shift. Rather it will widen the prevailing paradigm in scientific medical editing. No one who knows the recent history of clinical science and the importance of controlling variation through statistics, logic, and the other tools of contemporary scientific method would even consider discarding these important tools. Our best present methodological standards have come to stay, but they will no longer be the endpoints in editorial evaluation of articles for publication.

Thus increasingly editors will demand something more. These extra elements are already known but still appear irregularly even in the best articles and in the best journals. The problem is how to introduce them universally without making intolerable demands on the author or the reader.

Readers have their saturation point, even if it seems sometimes that they can absorb medical journals for 36–48 hours a day. On the whole the editors of the general medical journals recognise this problem better than those of the ever increasing number of special journals, whose authors and editors sometimes seem to forget the readers altogether and the problem of their time to read and think.

Leading general medical journals will have to remember the restrictions much more in future. They should try to ensure that the average reader spending one hour reading the journal each week will be guaranteed the necessary insight into major diagnostic, therapeutic, and preventive advances in general medicine. Furthermore, journals will have to introduce new combinations of printed and computerised text to let readers decide for themselves how to combine screening (retrieving) and close reading (deep digging). Structured abstracts seem to be the first step towards moving more details from a printed to a stored version. Even so, the condition remains that the stored part of the manuscript has been carefully edited. For the editors the workload of processing the rejected as well as the accepted, non-printed, articles will become so great that the traditional image of the hidden part of the iceberg will be an inadequate description.

Biomedical ethics will be another important issue to bear in mind when writing, editing, or reading medical journals. The special subgroup of medical ethics, research ethics, has already become a decisive factor in the decision to publish reports of experiments and studies in man. But others forms of ethics are rarely, or not at all, touched on in medical articles. The ethics of the distribution of health care and the questions of health sector priorities are often touched on in the public media and in editorial comments, but feature very rarely as an important part of an original scientific article. In future we must expect such new concepts to be introduced alongside the traditional ones about cost, efficacy, side effects, etc, thus enabling the reader to introduce a new technique into his clinical decision making. Articles on, for instance, a new artificial heart will have to include comments on whether such a new technique can be offered to all in need, within a fair and democratic health system, whether at the time of publication or in the foreseeable future.

Health resources have always been limited in relation to the potential of clinical medicine, but only recently have the scales started to fall from the eyes of our citizens, doctors, and politicians. Medical articles are still often written as if such things as a free lunch actually existed, or in a kind of economic vacuum, where money and other resources belong to a different world, and certainly not to the one of science and medicine. Many will argue against including economic aspects as part of a standard article format: costs will change, they will say, adding 'the more we use new methods, the cheaper they become.' My answer is that we must construct non-statistical confidence intervals for our health economic calculations just as we make so many other approximations in medical sciences and in clinical decision making.

Linguistic precision, readable style, and brevity will all be greater challenges than they are today. Confronted with this statement, many authors and editors will undoubtedly protest strongly, claiming that they already pay much attention to these aspects and have done so for years. Undoubtedly the language and style of medical journals have improved, especially so far as clarity is concerned. But language is not a central focus for many authors and editors. Young authors learn to produce the technical, anaemic, and tribalistic scientific language that they themselves find in journals, and which they expect editors to find most appropriate.

A large number of abbreviations sometimes makes reading similar to driving a car without shock absorbers. The best journals always explain them when the reader meets them for the first time. Clinical diagnoses are often presented as if there was an international consensus on every term, from migraine to ulcerative colitis, instead of giving brief definitions or references in the Methods section. Brevity is still a paramount necessity, especially if, as I expect, journals increasingly develop printed abstracts and computer retrievable background information.

Special problems exist in the English language journals because many authors do not have English as their mother tongue. Far from accepting any 'field chopper English', international journals ought to see English more and more as the international medical language and not God's gift to a few privileged countries. But even more important will be to strengthen all the curricula of medical schools: no more can we rely on present postgraduate self instruction in English, based on trial and error.

The copy editing tradition is efficient enough at removing mis-spellings and misconcepts but is insufficient as real style editing. Today the result is often to castrate the style and—at least in manuscripts from non-anglophone countries—to introduce unrecognisable statements.

The most important new constituent of a future editorial paradigm is undoubtedly an emphasis on reaching larger target groups. For every biomedical journal the core group of readers will be professionals working within a journal's discipline(s) together with those consumers of information outside their personal research subjects—that is, university teachers in medicine and clinicians. But what we often forget is the large group of secondary and tertiary readers (the terms do not reflect any ranking): nurses, midwives, physiotherapists, health administrators, health politicians, and newspaper and television journalists, together with the unhomogenous but important group—the thoughtful citizen.

All too often the style and language of medical journals are more exclusive than they need to be. Often hard scientific facts may be expressed differently, without losing scientific precision, and in this way could reach more unconditioned readers. It is not easy to change tradition and habits within medical writing, but the demand for a larger linguistic range ought to be part of any future editorial paradigm.

Conclusion

The era after randomised controlled trials will present editors with new challenges. Nevertheless, the future editorial paradigm will not be reached through revolution, but through evolution.

Editors and authors have the intellectual capacity to deal with the challenges, if only they learn from what takes place in society outside the health services and sciences. Here realignments of paradigms are well under way already.

1 Gosset WS ('Student'). On the probable error of the mean. *Biometrika* 1907;5:315.
2 Pearson K. Eighteen articles written in 1893–1912 about mathematical contributions to the theory of evolution. *Biometrika* 1901–36.
3 Fisher RA. *Statistical methods for research workers*. Edinburgh: Oliver & Boyd, 1925–54.
4 Hill AB. *Principles of medical statistics*, 49th ed. London: Lancet, 1971.
5 Witts LJ. *Medical surveys and clinical trials*. London: Oxford University Press, 1959.

Closing the gap between what researchers can do and what clinicians use: the journals' role

ROBERT H FLETCHER

A simple view of journal editors' work, which many scholars probably hold, is that editors sort out good manuscripts from bad ones, offending many good people along the way, then present unassailable articles in a respectable, convenient package, the hard copy journal. The rest should take care of itself: the articles will be read and used to change clinical practice. The latter steps are beyond the editors' control.

Of course, journal editing has never been so simple, and it is getting even less so. A number of forces in society, including specialisation in medicine, more complex research methods, and increased attention from the mass media and public at large are making editors' roles even more complex now. One of these forces is the increased attention to the end results of medical care.

What we all want—journal editors, authors, and readers alike— is for clinical research to improve medical care, and hence patients' health. This emphasis on outcomes, the end results of medical care, is certainly not new.[1] However, outcomes are receiving increasing attention recently. For example, the United States government has launched a new programme of grants specifically to assess the outcomes and costs of medical care.[2] Perhaps this new found interest is because society is more inclined to question everything, including the value of research and the relation between the process of medical care (what doctors do to and for patients) and the outcomes of care. There also is a growing awareness that even relatively

OPPORTUNITIES FOR JOURNALS TO
IMPROVE THE PROCESS

RESEARCH Publish articles about research methods
      Encourage teaching about methods in articles
      Set high standards for publication

ARTICLES Critique articles published in own journal
      Reviews by experts in research methods:
        External reviewers
        Own staff
      Methodological checklists

AVAILABLE Encourage innovations in disseminating information

SORTING Highlight scientific strengths and weaknesses of
      articles:
        In text
        In abstracts (structured abstracts)
      Publish collections of articles selected for scientific
      strength
      Publish meta-analyses, quantitative decision making

READ AND USED Improve attractiveness of presentation and format

BETTER PATIENT CARE

FIGURE—*Steps along the way from research to clinical practice: role of journals*

affluent countries cannot pay for all the services that patients would like to have and clinicians would like to give.

In this chapter I will consider the sequence of events from the development of excellent clinical research through publication to improved clinical decision making (figure). For each step, I will consider some of the factors that affect the transition to the next step and suggest some actions that journal editors might take to increase the chances of moving on to the next one. My remarks will concern original research published in peer reviewed medical journals for clinicians. I understand that these journals have many other functions;[3] [4] however, original research is their keystone.

My main point is that journal editors' opportunities to improve

109

medical care—indeed, their responsibilities—are broader than ever and that editors must find imaginative ways to meet these responsibilities. I understand that many editors, especially those of general medical journals, have already found ways to rise to this challenge. However, this aspect of editing has usually not been made explicit when editors have written about their work. I assume that we could meet these responsibilities better if we identified and discussed them directly.

Clinical research methods

There has been an extraordinary growth in the methods of clinical research, just as there has been in the laboratory sciences. Some of the new methods were imported from the work of epidemiologists and some were developed by clinicians themselves. Computers have helped, because the calculations necessary to accomplish some tasks— for example, the simultaneous adjustment for many variables that are unequally distributed between two groups, to make a fair comparison—simply were not possible before the development of modern computers. The predominance of chronic diseases in many countries has also encouraged the development of strong research methods; they pose intellectual challenges (for example, many variables acting in concert, long latency between cause and effect, and relatively small treatment effects) that require more powerful research methods.[5]

Developments in clinical research have prompted David Sackett to suggest that 'clinical epidemiology' (a term used for this these skills and perspectives) is a 'basic science for clinical medicine.'[6] Formal learning in this subject is increasingly popular[7], and represented by several textbooks,[5 6 8-11] national courses, research fellowships, and a renamed journal, the *Journal of Clinical Epidemiology*.

As a result of these developments there is a small but growing number of researchers who are scholars of clinical research methods themselves, rather than a biologically defined content area. They have studied the methods in the classroom, read about them, applied them under the attention of a mentor, and in other ways become experts. Most of them are young and many do not have subspecialty training. They are contributing much to the quality of clinical research. Most members of the medical research community, however, are much less interested and specialised in *clinical* research methods, and this must be taken into account when proposing solutions. They have learned clinical research methods on the job, often from a mentor who was not well versed in these methods.

Journals can help scholars in the research community as a whole to improve their grasp of advances in clinical research methods. Journals now publish teaching articles *about* research methods,[12-15] even though most of their readers are not researchers. Often the articles themselves are taken as an opportunity for small, relatively palatable teaching points about methods. Journals can also raise the level of clinical research by the standards they set for acceptance.

Quality of published research

How good is published clinical research, relative to basic criteria for scientific credibility? To be charitable, there is room for improvement.[16] Studies have shown that: clinical questions are addressed with relatively weak study designs[17]; sample size for most clinical trials is too small to detect confidently even relatively large, clinically important effects[18]; and clinical trials[19] and studies of diagnostic tests[20] often do not meet even basic standards for scientific validity.

Is the situation improving? We could find no evidence of improvement for articles published in 1946–76.[21] During that time the number of patients studied got smaller, strong designs more rare, and case reports remained the most common kind of study. But there is reason to believe that published clinical research has become stronger in the past decade. Well done clinical trials, case control studies, and the use of modern methods of controlling for extraneous variables seem to be more common recently. However, direct evidence supporting this belief is scarce. In one published report studies of diagnostic tests met more of a set of basic criteria for soundness in 1988 than in 1986.[22]

Journal editors can help to improve the research they publish in several ways. They can publish critiques of the scientific credibility of articles in their own journals, looking not at individual studies but at the pattern of strengths and weaknesses in the journal as a whole.[13 23] Editors can select reviewers who are experts in research methods, in addition to the usual experts in the content topic. Statistical reviewers on the editorial staff can assess research methods; however, few journals are large enough to afford this luxury. A methodological checklist, such as the one used by the *British Medical Journal*, is another means of quality control. If checklists are used, I hope they will be applied at the end of the review process, as at the beginning they might squelch some of the insights and perspectives of reviewers that are so valuable. With the assistance of external reviewers, editors teach authors, one at a time, about research methods through their correspondence; this teaching takes place whether or not the manuscripts are accepted for publication. Finally, journal editors can model humility and self criticism by carrying out research on their own decisions concerning peer review policies.[24]

All of these actions are to help improve the performance level of the research community as a whole over time. In the short term, a journal's contents cannot be made much better than the practice of research in the community of scholars that write for it. It is not feasible, in the time available, to raise standards for publication much further.

Availability

In a technical sense, published research is widely available and rapidly becoming more so. *Index Medicus* in hard copy has been followed by the availability of citations and abstracts in libraries via telephone lines, then direct to individuals using their own microcomputers. CD-ROM technology now removes the need for telephone lines, a major obstacle in developing countries. Electronic publishing is also becoming more complete: first there were just abstracts, then full text and tables, and recently figures too.

There is, of course, the usual delay from when the technology is available until clinicians use it. At the present time, most of the world's doctors, even in developed countries, do not have peer reviewed research articles readily available to them on a day to day basis. The literature will almost certainly be more available as time passes. The change will probably be much slower than it seems it should be. But it is not the technology, or even the cost, that holds readers back.

Sorting

The real problem in making information available to clinicians is, ironically, the very wealth and availability of information. For most clinical questions, there are far more articles than one can read, and many of them are not much good. They need to be sorted in two ways: by content, which is readily available now, and by scientific strength, which is not.

For example, suppose I want to find out for myself, from the original research reports, about the clinical usefulness of carcinoembryonic antigen, a blood test for cancer. I can easily obtain citations for most of the world's published reports using my personal computer. There are many thousands of them.[25] Restricting the search—for example, to articles about diagnosis—will help me narrow the field, but many articles (thousands) will remain. They are published in hundreds of journals and are of every conceivable level of quality. I cannot read them all, and I want the best. I can enter methods terms into the search which may also improve the specificity of my search although at the penalty of a decreased sensitivity of unknown magnitude. The technology has not, so far, helped me much.

There is another limitation in making unselected articles available. Most readers are not well prepared to distinguish the good from the bad. These skills are not generally taught in medical school, not reinforced in postgraduate training, and not just 'picked up' informally.[26]

Journals can help their readers over this barrier in at least three ways. Firstly, they can highlight the scientific strengths and weaknesses of each original research study they publish, in the text and by means of structured abstracts.[27] Secondly, they can publish collections of abstracts that have been selected by experts for their scientific strength and clinical usefulness. The American College of Physicians is planning to publish such a collection, a supplement to the *Annals of Internal Medicine* called *ACP Journal Club*, beginning next year. We are indebted to Brian Haynes, who will edit this new publication. Thirdly, journals can publish more articles that include sorting and weighing as an essential element. Meta-analysis[28] and quantitative decision making[29] make these processes explicit, and so are a step forward from more traditional, narrative reviews.

Using the best

As the saying goes, 'you can lead a horse to water but you cannot make him drink.' Probably the biggest obstacle to overcome, if clinicians are to use the best published research in their practices, is to somehow attract them to good articles in good journals. There is evidence that journals are only one of many sources of information for clinicians.[30] The competition among journals themselves is formidable. Apparently the tradition and prestige of peer reviewed journals do not always assure their success in the competition. 'Throwaway' journals are extremely successful, at least in the US. If advertisements are a way to judge readership (and many businesses have bet their future on it) then journals publishing peer reviewed, original research have a humble place in physicians' reading habits. Only two such journals are in the top 10 in advertisement sales in the US; the highest ranked stands behind *Medical Economics*.[31]

It is not difficult to guess some of the reasons that other sources of information are so popular. Physicians are very busy and easily overwhelmed by all the information they should master. They need practical, attractive ways of keeping up. Moreover, 'throwaway' journals make every effort to make their message attractive. There is a dark side to this: over simplifying the message, playing down uncertainty, and soliciting articles on popular (not necessarily important) topics are not good for the practice of medicine. But there are also lessons for peer reviewed journals. The presentation and format are more attractive. Many prestigious journals have taken a certain amount of pride in their relatively drab format: muted colours, small print, dull but orderly tables, and the like. Maybe they can learn something valuable from the 'throwaways' about attractiveness without sacrificing quality.[32]

Summary

As the complexity of medical information grows, editors should take responsibility for more aspects of the medical information system as a whole, especially the use of strong research methods, ways of helping clinicians sort out published reports according to scientific strength, and making the good publications more attractive to an easily distracted audience. In doing this, journals will be fostering their real mission, to improve the health and medical care of the people.

1 Codman EA. A study of hospital efficiency as represented by the product. *Tr Am Gynec Soc* 1914;**39**:60–100.
2 Medical treatment effectiveness research program described. *Research Activities* 1990;**127**:3. (Department of Health and Human Services, Public Health Services)
3 Lock S. *A difficult balance: editorial peer review in medicine*. Philadelphia: ISI Press, 1986.
4 Fletcher RH, Fletcher SW. A transition. *Ann Intern Med* 1990;**113**:6–8.
5 Fletcher RH, Fletcher SW, Wagner EH. *Clinical epidemiology. The essentials*. Baltimore: Williams and Wilkins, 1988.
6 Sackett DL, Haynes RB, Tugwell P. *Clinical epidemiology. A basic science for clinical medicine*. Boston: Little Brown, 1985.
7 Fletcher RH, Fletcher SW. Clinical epidemiology. A new science for an old art. *Ann Intern Med* 1983;**99**:401–3.
8 Feinstein AR. *Clinical epidemiology. The architecture of clinical research*. Philadelphia: WB Saunders, 1985.
9 Weis N. *Clinical epidemiology. Study of the natural history of disease*. New York: Oxford University Press, 1986.
10 Jenicek M, Cleroux R. *Epidemiologie clinique*. St-Hyacinthe, Quebec:Edisem,1985.

114

11 Kramer MS. *Clinical epidemiology and biostatistics. A primer for clinical investigators and decision-makers.* New York:Springer,1988.

12 Sackett DL. (Department of Clinical Epidemiology and Biostatistics, McMaster University Health Sciences Centre.) How to read clinical journals. I. Why to read them and how to start reading them critically. *Can Med Assoc J* 1981;**124**:555–90.

13 Bailar JC III, Mosteller F. *Medical uses of statistics.* Boston, Massachusetts:NEJM Books,1986.

14 Research Development Committee, Society for Research and Education in Primary Care Internal Medicine. Clinical research methods: an annotated bibliography. *Ann Intern Med* 1983;**99**:419–24.

15 Gardner MJ, Altman DG. *Statistics with confidence.* London:BMJ Books,1989.

16 Williamson JW, Goldschmidt PG, Colton T. The quality of medical literature: an analysis of validation assessments. In: Bailor JC, Mosteller F, eds. *Medical uses of statistics.* Waltham, Massachusetts:NEJM Books,1986.

17 Fletcher SW, Fletcher RH, Greganti MA. Clinical research trends in general medical journals: questions addressed, phenomena measured and research designs used from 1946 to 1976. EB Roberts, RI Levy, SN Finkelstein, J Moscowitz, EJ Sondik, eds. In: *Proceedings of Conference on the Development and Dissemination of Biomedical Innovations.* Cambridge, Massachusetts:MIT Press,1981.

18 Friedman JA, Chalmers TC, Smith H Jr, Kuebler RR. The importance of beta, the type II error and sample size in the design and interpretation of the randomized control trial. *N Engl J Med* 1978;**299**:690–4.

19 Mosteller F, Gilbert JP, McPeek B. Reporting standards and research strategies for controlled trials. Agenda for the editor. *Controlled Clin Trials* 1980;**1**:37–58.

20 Sheps SB, Schechter MT. The assessment of diagnostic tests: a survey of current medical research. *JAMA* 1984;**252**:2418–22.

21 Fletcher RH. Clinical research in general medical journals. A 30 year perspective. *N Engl J Med* 1979;**301**:180–3.

22 Arroll B, Schecter MT, Sheps SB. *J Gen Intern Med 1988*;**3**:443–7.

23 Cooper GS, Zangwill L. An analysis of the quality of research reports in the Journal of General Internal Medicine. *J Gen Intern Med* 1989;**4**:232–6.

24 Guarding the guardians. Research on editorial peer review. *JAMA* 1990;**263**:1317–1438 (entire issue).

25 Fletcher RH. Carcinoembryonic antigen. *Ann Intern Med* 1986;**104**:66–73.

26 Fletcher RH. Three ways of knowing in clincial medicine. *South Med J* 1990;**83**:308–12.

27 Haynes RB, Mulrow CD, Huth EJ, Altman DG, Gardner MJ. More informative abstracts revisited. *Ann Intern Med* 1990;**113**:69–76.

28 L'Abbe KA, Detsky AS, O'Rourke K. Meta-analysis in clinical research. *Ann Intern Med* 1987;**107**:224–33.

29 Sox HC Jr, Blatt MA, Higgens MC, Marton KI. *Medical decision making.* Boston:Butterworth,1988.

30 Williamson JW, German PS, Weiss R, Skinner EA, Bowes F III. Health science information management and continuing education of physicians. A survey of US primary care practitioners and their opinion leaders. *Ann Intern Med* 1989; **110**:151–60.

31 *Medical Marketing and Media* 1990 (March):30.

32 Rennie D, Bero LA. Throw it away, Sam. The controlled circulation journals. *CBE Views* 1990;**1**:31–5.

How clinical journals could serve clinician readers better

R BRIAN HAYNES

Medical practitioners suffer from information problems that lead to declining clinical competence as time passes from formal training. Most practitioners prefer to keep up to date by reading clinical journals. From a clinical perspective, however, clinical journals serve a meagre fare that consists of too little nourishment to sustain clinical competence and too much that is potentially toxic to patient care. Though clinical journals cannot be blamed for more than a part of the information problems of clinicians, they could take a leadership role in helping solve some of these problems. In this chapter I shall describe some of the pertinent information needs of doctors and ways in which journals interested in serving clinical audiences better might help.

Problems of doctors in using the biomedical literature

Doctors have two complementary information needs that could be aided by clinical journals: news and details of genuine advances in health care as they occur (current awareness) and access to the best information on specific medical problems as these problems arise in clinical practice (problem solving). For current awareness, studies have documented considerable delays and errors in the clinical implementation of validated findings from health care research after they are reported in published biomedical reports.[1] [2] The extent to which doctors are aware of current standards of clinical practice is strongly negatively correlated with the length of time that they have been in practice.[3] This does not appear to be for lack of effort to keep up to date. Most practitioners state that they read medical journals two to three hours a week and that this is their preferred means of keeping up to date.[4-7] At face value, this may seem like a large commitment to continuing education in general and to journal reading in particular. However, it must be recalled that over 75 000 articles are published in biomedical journals each week[8] and that publications relating to a given specialty are scattered widely. Indeed, Weiner and his colleagues reported that only 15% of original articles on the risk of breast cancer from oral contraceptives appeared in specialist journals for obstetrics and gynecology, and likened this situation to a form of censorship, denying specialists in obstetrics and gynecology access to primary data.[9] Extracting the publications that are relevant to a given clinical question is time consuming and is made even more difficult by the facts that many studies at all stages are flawed[10-12] or reported misleadingly.[13-15]

As for problem solving, doctors state that they are overwhelmed by the biomedical literature.[16] They lack time and do not know where to look when they require information.[17] As a result they very seldom attempt to use journal articles to seek information on the problems of individual patients.[17] However, clinicians are turning increasingly to electronic searching of published medical reports to solve problems.[16 18]

Ways clinical journals can increase their clinical utility

The problems that doctors have in using clinical journals are not surprising: the biomedical literature is best suited to scientists, not clinical practitioners.[19] From a practice perspective, clinical journals could help in many ways: increasing their allegiance to clinical practitioners, organising articles according to the maturity of investigations, presenting information from studies more accurately, innovating and testing ways to improve article selection and information communication, and customising information for the solution of clinical problems.

ALLEGIANCE

The articles that appear in peer reviewed clinical journals indicate that the allegiance of clinical journals is much more to scientists than to clinicians. Most articles report studies that are too preliminary for clinical use: laboratory studies (including physiological studies among humans), case reports, uncontrolled field studies, and poorly designed trials.[20] These studies are crucial to the advance

117

of science but can be misleading if their findings are incorporated too early into clinical practice. Thus, preliminary studies are better suited to communication from scientist to scientist than from scientist to clinician.[21] The reasons for publishing these preliminary studies in clinical journals are doubtless complex but probably include: too few sound studies to fill the quota of journal pages, mistaking the importance of the clinical problems that these articles address with the importance of the information in the studies for solving the problem, and perhaps the failure of journal editors and reviewers to distinguish definitive studies about clinical problems from studies that are not.

It would not be of concern that clinical journals serve scientists better than clinicians were it not that clinicians need journals that help them keep up to date and that clinical journals are supported largely by subscriptions paid by clinicians and advertising revenues from companies seeking the attention of clinicians. Under these conditions, clinical journals could well justify working hard to ensure that clinicians are presented with the best studies and reviews suited to immediate clinical application. If there are not enough such articles to fill journal pages, clinicians would not object if the frequency of publication were reduced or the number of journals competing for the same clincial audience were cut down. There are probably enough advanced studies in each major specialty of medicine for one or two journals to flourish on studies from the final stages of testing clinical innovations, augmented by systematic overviews on important clinical topics. Journals that wished to enhance their relevance to clinical practice could position themselves by stating this policy for contributors and, when articles are selected for publication, by giving preference to studies designed to answer clinical questions direct.*

Because clinical journals have not evolved in this way, there are now a large number of glitzy 'throwaway' journals that compete for the reading time of practitioners by offering practitioners exactly what they want: clinically oriented information. There is nothing wrong with this if we accept that clinicians do not need to see primary sources when they are published, that paying authors for their contributions is an adequate substitute for peer review, and that corporate sponsorship of these publications will not influence

---

* I am tempted to use the term 'clinical research' here but this was coopted long ago by laboratory researchers doing preliminary studies among humans.

Basic standards for studies of direct importance to clinical practice

Study purpose	Design criterion
All studies	Outcome measure of clinical importance
Prognosis	Recruitment of an inception cohort of individuals who are intially free of the outcome being studied
Diagnosis	Independent (blind) comparison of test and of criterion standard of diagnosis
Prevention, treatment	Intervention and control groups formed by random allocation
Aetiology	Comparison of groups exposed and not exposed to the putative causal factor, with statistical adjustment for confounding factors
Review study	Indication of the sources of articles and the criteria for selecting articles for review

which authors are invited to contribute or what information is presented.

ORGANISING ARTICLES ACCORDING TO MATURITY

Many clinical journals place what they consider to be the most important articles at the front of each issue, perhaps after editorials. This could suit clinicians well if what journal editors chose as important is based on suitability for immediate clinical application. Unfortunately, most journals mix preliminary studies with more mature investigations, the choice of importance apparently based on a mixture of originality, importance of the clinical problem, scientific merit, newsworthiness, and, probably, luck of the draw. Alternatively, all original investigations are lumped together, regardless of the stage of testing they represent.

Clinicans would be served better if journals would put the most definitive investigations for clinical practice in a prominent, separate, location in each issue. Selection of such articles on methodological grounds need not be difficult; the basic standards appear in the table. Review studies (systematic overviews) on clinical topics that meet basic criteria for scientific rigour would also appear in such a section. If no studies published in an issue meet these criteria, it would be most helpful if editors would keep the section heading on the contents page and indicate that no studies met the criteria. Although editors may find this suggestion outlandish, I do not believe that clinicians would. This approach might also help the lay press in its reporting, reducing exaggerated interpretations of preliminary findings.

PRESENTATION OF INFORMATION IN ARTICLES

Whether or not journals wish to cater more to clinical practitioners, clinicians (and scientists) would be helped by improvements in the standards of reporting. Surveys of published reports have documented distressingly high rates of errors of omission and commission in methodology, statistics, quotations, citations, and conclusions.[11] [15] [22] [23] The adoption of uniform requirements for manuscripts submitted to biomedical journals has been a major advance in medical publishing,[24] particularly for specifying key methodological details in the conduct and analysis of studies. These requirements are quite comprehensive for original studies but require further interpretation if they are to be followed by authors. Bailar and Mosteller have provided clarifications for statistical procedures and reporting,[25] but these need be incorporated into instructions for authors so that they are available when manuscripts are prepared. The uniform requirements also need to be augmented with standards for review articles[26] [27] and for more informative abstracts.[28] [29]

Many journals require authors to submit manuscripts according to the uniform requirements, and a growing number ask authors to follow the guidelines for abstracts of original articles and systematic reviews[29], but the process for checking and ensuring adherence needs to be bolstered. Gardner and Bond have provided preliminary evidence of the value of formal statistical review,[30] and journals would do well to emulate this lead. The editor of the *Canadian Medical Association Journal* has recently prepared guidelines for authors and reviewers that may help in ensuring adherence by making the criteria explicit and by incorporating them formally into the review process.[31–35]

Of particular concern is accuracy in the reporting of conclusions. The uniform requirements state: 'avoid unqualified statements and conclusions not completely supported by your data', but this is often ignored[23]. Though scientists can be expected to recognise such deviations, clinicians may take short cuts, looking only for conclusions. For this reason, the impact of the requirements would be greatly strengthened if journal editors and reviewers insisted on fidelity from authors in stating their conclusions in a succinct and non-speculative way, in both the abstract and the discussion section. Conclusions should not stray beyond the evidence presented, and important negative conclusions must not be omitted from either the abstract or the text.

INNOVATING AND TESTING

There have been several innovations in journal publication over the decades, including the uniform requirements and the recent reformatting of several major journals. However, the First International Congress on Peer Review in Biomedical Publication held in 1989, showed just how little research and evaluation has been done on the process of selecting and processing articles for publication.[36] What limited evidence was presented indicated extensive variability in the way in which peer review was conducted,[37] in the consistency of ratings by reviewers,[38] and in the fidelity of detecting errors.[23][30] It seems ironic that the process of reporting science is so unscientific. There is hope for the future, however. Certainly, the improvement in standards for reporting methods and results, embodied in the uniform requirements, is an advance. The move to explicit criteria for peer review is in keeping with the best scientific standards for improving the reliability of subjective measurements. The new capsular comments in the table of contents of *Annals of Internal Medicine* may help readers to be selective with minimal effort—but only if these 'ultraterse communications'[8] are precisely accurate conclusions from the studies they represent. Recalling the inaccuracies of authors' conclusions,[15][22] this may simply magnify an unsolved problem. Similarly, the highlights at the beginning of the *British Medical Journal* may help readers to be selective—but clinical readers will not be served well if these 'terse communications' are not based on clinical priorities.

Formal evaluations are required to assess whether these innovations have hit their targets. Clinical journals also need to do research into their readers' needs and to develop innovations to serve these needs. The current use by journals of crude circulation figures, citation counts, and impact factors to calculate success is inadequate and misleading. Circulation is an artificial measure for most major journals, with captive, membership audiences. Scientists, not clinicians, cite articles in print. To do a better job, journals will need to spend part of their time and other resources for innovation and testing. The revenues from clinical journals are possibly being diverted into other activities of the organisations that sponsor them or the corporations that own them. Though these funds are no doubt being put to good use, channelling money into innovation and research may well pay bigger dividends. If improvements in clinical journals led to increased readership and increased impact on readers, subscription and advertising revenues would rise. If jour-

121

nals do not currently have the expertise or staff to do much research and development, perhaps affiliating with the growing number of university medical informatics programmes would help.[39]

CUSTOMISING INFORMATION TO SOLVE CLINICAL PROBLEMS

Most of the foregoing proposals are aimed at improving the value of clinical journals for the current awareness of doctors. There is an even greater need to organise journal articles to help doctors solve clinical problems. Clinicians must be able to retrieve, in a matter of minutes, the best information published on a given problem. Thumbing through journals is not likely to produce the needed information and using a given journal is problematic when the information could be in any one of so many.

Textbooks have traditionally provided information for solving clinical problems, but textbooks cannot keep pace with the journal publication of new information. For example early in 1990 neither of the current editions of the two most popular medical texts in North America[40][41] indicated the lifesaving properties of enalapril for severe congestive heart failure three years after this was reported in the *New England Journal of Medicine*[42]. Regularly updated texts such as Scientific American *Medicine*[43] and specialised compendia such as the *Oxford Database of Perinatal Trials*[44] can overcome this problem, but there are too few of these at present to cover more than a fraction of the problems of medical practice. Meanwhile doctors are turning increasingly to self service, electronic searches of medical published reports.[16][18]

Journals could foster and enhance the clinical use of electronic access to publications in several ways. Firstly, the numbers and skills of doctors using electronic services, though increasing rapidly, could be improved by articles in journals on the value of and techniques for clinical problem solving. Secondly, the indexing of journal articles in MEDLINE remains an important barrier to the effectiveness and efficiency of electronic searching.[45][46] Journals could work with authors to promote and improve keywording and with the electronic services to improve indexing. Thirdly, the amount and accuracy of information in titles and abstracts in the bibliographic databases are less than desirable, and journals should be devoting more thought and resources to perfecting these two essential parts of their articles. Structured abstracts were developed to provide clinicians with more information on which to assess the validity and applicability of journal articles for clinical practice,[29] and journals should be using these if they wish their articles to be represented best in terms of both accuracy and details. (For example, the US National Library of Medicine truncates abstracts at 250 words for articles less than 10 pages long *unless* the abstract is structured.) Finally, full text journal databases are an important complement to bibliographic databases but have been slow to develop for several reasons that can be circumvented if the current leading clinical journals (many of which are already represented in the BRS COLLEAGUE full text database) were able to provide a high concentration of clinically relevant literature and if the technical problems of representing tables and figures were overcome. The latter problem may be overcome by compact disk, a medium which journal editors should be exploring with vigour.

Finally, clinical journals could be seeking out and collaborating with third parties, including professional societies, universities, and publishers, in developing and disseminating sound derivative information services that address the information needs of specific clinical disciplines. The products of these joint ventures would be current awareness periodicals that are precisely tailored to the users' needs, medical literature databases that synthesise evidence from studies about clinical problems and that are constantly updated, and the timely incorporation of genuine advances in medical knowledge into quality assurance activities. Though clinical journals may not play the leading role in these innovations, the articles they publish are the key to the success of the innovations, and journals can be very active partners in this process.

Discussion

Many of these suggestions for clinical journals may be challenged as impractical. For example, the proposal that journals increase the concentration of definitive studies by advertising to attract more such studies and discouraging the submission of articles from preliminary investigations might be felt to threaten the options and stability of journals. What if authors of articles on preliminary studies heeded the new directions but authors of advanced clinical investigations did not? The increase in clinical subscriptions that would probably result if a journal adopted this policy (or even advertised that it was implementing it) would make this prospect unlikely. So, too, would increased circulation obviate the fear that reducing the frequency of publication might be committing financial suicide. If clinicians had an easier time of extracting relevant and valid information from clinical journals, more might subscribe,

123

more companies might advertise, and revenues might actually increase despite the decreasing volume of publication. My guess is that there are enough well designed and executed clinicial studies and well conducted literature overviews to support one or more clinical journals in most clinical disciplines. The first journals that adopt a policy of tailoring their publications for clinicians might do very well indeed. But the financial implications have not been studied. Nor can they be until some brave journals test the waters. This is not to say that the process of changing to suit clinical information needs is all or none. All journals that seek to help scientists disseminate and clinicians keep up with important advances in health care may find at least some of the proposals worth pursuing.

1 Stross JK, Harlan WR. The dissemination of new medical information. *JAMA* 1979;**241**:2662–4.
2 Lomas J, Haynes RB. A taxonomy and critical review of tested strategies for the application of clinical practice recommendations: from 'official' to 'individual' clinical policy. *Am J Prev Med* 1988;**4** (suppl 2):77–94.
3 Evans CE, Haynes RB, Birkett NR, Gilbert JR, Taylor DW, Sackett DL, *et al.* Does a mailed continuing education program improve physician performance? Results of a randomized trial. *JAMA* 1986;**255**:501–4.
4 Curry L, Putnam W. Continuing education in Maritime Canada: the methods physicians use, would prefer, and find most effective. *Can Med Assoc J* 1981;**124**: 563–6.
5 Currie BF. Continuing education from medical periodicals. *J Med Educ* 1976;**51**: 420.
6 Stinson ER, Mueller DA. Survey of health professionals' information needs and habits. *JAMA* 1980;**243** 140–3.
7 Council on Medical Education. Survey of the current status of continuing medical education. *Association American College of Continuing Medical Education Newsletter* 1981;**10**:2–20.
8 Bernier CL, Yerkey AN. *Cogent communication*. Westport, Connecticut: Greenwood Press, 1979:39.
9 Weiner JM, Shirley S, Gilman NJ, Stowe SM, Wolf RM. Access to data and the information explosion: oral contraceptives and the risk of cancer. *Contraception* 1981;**24**:301–13.
10 Fletcher RH, Fletcher SW. Clinical research in general medical journals: a 30 year perspective. *N Engl J Med* 1979;**301**:180–3.
11 Cooper GS, Zangwill L. An analysis of the quality of research reports in the *Journal of General Internal Medicine*. *J Gen Intern Med* 1989;**4**:232–6.
12 DerSimonian R, Charette LJ, McPeek B, Mosteller F. Reporting on methods in clinical trials. *N Engl J Med* 1982;**306**:1332–7.
13 Bailar JC 3rd, Louis TA, Lavori PW, Polansky M. A classification for biomedical research reports. *N Engl J Med* 1984;**311**:1482–7.
14 Bailar JC 3rd. Science, statistics, and deception. *Ann Intern Med* 1986;**104**:259–60.
15 Gotzsche P. Methodology and overt and hidden bias in reports of 196 double-blind trials of nonsteroidal antiinflammatory drugs in rheumatoid arthritis. *Controlled Clin Trials* 1989;**10**:31–56.

124

16 Williamson JW, German PS, Weiss R, Skinner EA, Bowes F III. Health science information management and continuing education of physicians. *Ann Intern Med* 1989;**110**:151–60.

17 Covell DG, Uman GC, Manning PR. Information needs in office practice: are they being met? *Ann Intern Med* 1985;**103**:596–9.

18 Haynes RB, McKibbon KA, Walker CJ, Ryan C, Fitzgerald D, Ramsden MF. Online access to MEDLINE in clinical settings. A study of use and usefulness. *Ann Intern Med* 1990;**112**:78–84.

19 Weiner JM, Shirley S, Gilman NJ, Stowe SM, Wolf RM. Access to data and the information explosion: oral contraceptives and the risk of cancer. *Contraception* 1981;**24**:301–13.

20 Fletcher RH, Fletcher SW. Clinical research in general medical journals. *N Engl J Med* 1979;**301**:180–3.

21 Haynes RB. Loose connections between peer reviewed clinical journals and clinical practice. *Ann Intern Med* 1990;**113**:724–8.

22 Evans M, Pollock AV. Trials on trial. A review of trials of antibiotic prophylaxis. *Arch Surg* 1984;**119**:109–13.

23 Evans JT. Nadjari HI, Burchell SA. Quotational and reference accuracy in surgical journals. A continuing peer review problem. *JAMA* 1990;**263**:1353–4.

24 International Committee of Medical Journal Editors. Uniform requirements for manuscripts submitted to biomedical journals. *Ann Intern Med* 1988;**108**:258–65.

25 Bailar JC, Mosteller F. Guidelines for statistical reporting in articles for medical journals. Amplifications and explanations. *Ann Intern Med* 1988;**108**:266–73.

26 Oxman AD, Guyatt GH. Guidelines for reading literature reviews. *Can Med Assoc J* 1988;**138**:697–703.

27 Mulrow C. The medical review article: state of the science. *Ann Intern Med* 1987;**106**:484–7.

28 Ad hoc working group for critical appraisal of the medical literature (R B Haynes, chairman). A proposal for more informative abstracts of clinical articles. *Ann Intern Med* 1987;**106**:598–604.

29 Haynes RB, Mulrow CD, Huth EJ, Altman DG, Gardner MJ. More informative abstracts revisited: a progress report. *Ann Intern Med* 1990;**113**:69–76.

30 Gardner MJ, Bond J. An explanatory study of statistical assessment of papers published in the *British Medical Journal*. *JAMA* 1990;**263**:1355–7.

31 Squires BP. Descriptive studies: what editors want from authors and peer reviewers [editorial]. *Can Med Assoc J* 1989;**141**:879–80.

32 Squires BP. Case reports: what editors want from authors and peer reviewers [editorial]. *Can Med Assoc J* 1989;**141**:379–80.

33 Squires BP. Biomedical review articles: what editors want from authors and peer reviewers [editorial]. *Can Med Assoc J* 1989;**141**:195–7.

34 Squires BP. Biomedical manuscripts: what editors want from authors and peer reviewers [editorial]. *Can Med Assoc J* 1989;**141**:17–9.

35 Squires BP. Clarifying requirements for manuscripts [editorial]. *Can Med Assoc J* 1988;**138**:305–6.

36 Rennie D. Editorial peer review in biomedical publication. The first international congress [editorial]. *JAMA* 1990;**263**:1317.

37 Hargens LL. Variations in journal peer review systems. *JAMA* 1990;**263**:1348–52.

38 Garfunkel JM, Ulshen MH, Hamrick HJ, Lawson EE. Problems identified by secondary review of accepted manuscripts. *JAMA* 1990;**263**:1369–71.

39 American Association of Medical Colleges. Evaluation of medical information science in medical education. *J Med Educ* 1986;**61**:487–543.

40 J B Wyngaarden, L H Smith Jr, eds. *Cecil textbook of medicine*. 18th ed. Philadelphia: Saunders, 1988.

41 *Harrison's principles of internal medicine*. 11th ed. New York: McGraw-Hill, 1987.

42 The CONSENSUS Trial Study Group. Effects of enalapril on mortality in severe

congestive heart failure: results of the Cooperative North Scandinavian Enalapril Survival Study (CONSENSUS). *N Engl J Med* 1987;**316**:1429.

43 Rubenstein E, Federman DD, eds. Scientific American *Medicine*. (Discstest computer file.) New York: Scientific American 1989.

44 Chalmers I, ed. *Oxford database of perinatal trials* (software). New York: Oxford University Press, regularly updated.

45 Dickersin K, Hewitt P, Mutch L, Chalmers I, Chalmers TC. Perusing the literature: comparison of MEDLINE searching with a perinatal trials database. *Controlled Clin Trials* 1985;**6**:306–17.

46 Kirpalani H, Schmidt B, McKibbon KA, Haynes RB, Sinclair JC. Searching MEDLINE for high quality studies on care of the newborn. *Pediatrics* 1989;**83**:543–6.

Improving the quality and dissemination of reviews of clinical research

IAIN CHALMERS

If, as is sometimes supposed, science consisted in nothing but the laborious accumulation of facts, it would soon come to a standstill, crushed, as it were, under its own weight. The suggestion of a new idea, or the detection of a law, supersedes much that has previously been a burden on the memory, and by introducing order and coherence facilitates the retention of the remainder in an available form . . . Two processes are thus at work side by side, the reception of new material and the digestion and assimilation of the old; and as both are essential, we may spare ourselves the discussion of their relative importance.

Lord Rayleigh, 1884

The science of reviewing evidence

The words with which this chapter opens are taken from an address to the British Association for the Advancement of Science more than a century ago.[1] In his comments, Lord Rayleigh was urging scientists to recognise the importance of synthesising evidence derived from distinct but related investigations, so that any coherence among the results could be identified efficiently.

To judge from the behaviour of scientists and the institutions of science during the subsequent century, Lord Rayleigh's injunction has not been taken very seriously. The scientific community continues to have a remarkably casual attitude to the process of synthesising research evidence.[2] As Pillemer has put it, the usual approach is 'subjective, relying on idiosyncratic judgments about such key issues as which studies to include and how to draw overall conclusions. Studies are considered one at a time, with strengths and weaknesses selectively identified and casually discussed. Since the process is informal, it is not surprising that different reviewers often draw very different conclusions from the same set of studies'.[3]

During the past decade, this lack of interest in the science of reviewing evidence has become a matter for comment within the social scientific and biomedical fields.[4-10] As Kass noted in 1981 in Warren's seminal book on coping with the biomedical literature, 'reviews will need to be evaluated as critically as are primary scientific papers'.[5] Within the biomedical field, it was Mulrow who began the process foreseen by Kass. In an important article published in the *Annals of Internal Medicine* in 1987, Mulrow reported her assessment of the quality of the review articles published in four major medical journals, and concluded that current medical reviews do not usually use scientific methods to identify, assess, and synthesise information.[11] Since Mulrow's findings were published, others have noted how clinical scientists often seem to abandon scientific principles when reviewing evidence.[12-18]

Because medical practitioners place heavy reliance on reviews as a way of trying to deal with the information overload that confronts them,[19] continued tolerance of reviews that disregard scientific principles may well be reflected in adverse effects on patients. If this risk is to be reduced, the clinical research community, including editors, must make greater efforts to ensure that scientific principles are brought to bear on the review process.[12 15]

In the same way that steps must be taken to control bias and imprecision in conducting primary research, so also must precautions be taken to avoid these problems during the process of reviewing a body of evidence derived from a number of independently reported studies. As in other aspects of scientific activity, presenting the methodological details of reviews allows the study to be replicated. Different reviewers using the same materials and methods should arrive at similar conclusions. Others may disagree with the materials and methods used in a particular analysis; but at least they will know what was done, and they will have the opportunity to present an alternative analysis for consideration.[3]

Oxman and Guyatt have offered guidelines (summarised in table I) to help readers to assess the likely validity of a review article,[15] and Mulrow and her colleagues have suggested ways of preparing more informative abstracts of these articles.[20]

TABLE I — *Guidelines for assessing research reviews, reproduced from Oxman and Guyatt, 1988*[15]

Were the questions and methods clearly stated?
Were comprehensive search methods used to locate relevant studies?
Were explicit methods used to determine which articles to include in the review?
Was the validity of the primary studies assessed?
Was the assessment of primary studies reproducible and free from bias?
Was any variation in the findings of the relevant studies analysed?
Were the findings of the primary studies combined appropriately?
Were the conclusions of the reviewer(s) supported by the data cited?

Reducing random error by formal synthesis of data derived from distinct but related investigations

Wider application of scientific principles in reviewing evidence should help to reduce systematic errors (biases). In addition, random errors can be reduced by using appropriate statistical methods to integrate the results of distinct but related investigations, and this process is often an important component of formal reviews of evidence.

Informal assimilation and synthesis of the numerical data generated by a body of independent but related research studies will always be difficult, and will often be impossible.[13] This limitation of informal reviews has been demonstrated in both observational and experimental studies.[21][22] These have shown that important associations are sometimes overlooked when informal methods of review are used, but identified correctly when more systematic methods are applied. Statisticians have been using methods to synthesise evidence derived from a set of similar, but independent, investigations for at least half a century.[23] Although social, psychological, and medical researchers first used these methods more than 30 years ago,[24-26] a decade passed before they began to be adopted more widely.[27] During the 1970s, quantitative synthesis of research results was adopted rapidly by educational and psychological researchers, one of whom named the process 'meta-analysis'.[28]

There is no reason, in principle, why the methods used to achieve quantitative syntheses of the results of separate studies should not be applied to studies across the whole spectrum of clinical research (ranging from studies of aetiology and prognosis, through evaluations of screening and diagnostic tests, to assessments of the effects of interventions designed to prevent or treat disease). Although the process has been applied to studies using observational data (such as the study by Longnecker *et al*),[29] however, clinical researchers have mainly adopted meta-analysis to synthesise data derived from randomised clinical experiments.

Referring specifically to randomised trials, Peto has described the rationale for synthesising the results of similar but separate studies in meta-analyses (also referred to as 'overviews', or 'pooled analyses'): 'While we cannot assume that different trials are exactly comparable, or that patients in different trials are exactly comparable, it is reasonable to assume that if different trials address related questions then there is going to be some tendency for the answers to come out in the same direction. That tendency may well be obscured in individual trials, or even in some cases reversed, by the play of chance. But elsewhere it may remain, and it is that tendency which the overview is trying to detect.'[30]

Using meta-analyses of controlled trials to guide clinical practice and research

GUIDING CLINICAL PRACTICE

Because meta-analysis can help to reduce both incorrect acceptance and incorrect rejection of the null hypothesis (type I and type II errors), meta-analyses of the results of similar but distinct controlled trials can provide evidence which should enable clinicians and patients to make better treatment decisions. For example, some obstetricians and paediatricians believe that any beneficial effects on the incidence of neonatal respiratory distress which may result from administering corticosteroids to women who are expected to deliver preterm are confined to black, female babies born between 32 and 34 weeks gestation, and delivered more than 24 hours and less than seven days after the drug has been administered.[31] These biologically implausible views have resulted from type I errors made when data dredging within subgroups in particular trials has yielded 'statistically significant' differences between steroid and control groups. These false inferences might have been avoided if the authors of the reports of the individual trials had resisted the temptation to fish among subgroups for statistically significant differences. Even if investigators had been unable to resist this temptation, however, they and reviewers of this body of evidence would have avoided misleading their readers if they had used meta-analysis to integrate the results of a particular trial with the results of other, similar trials.[32]

Obstetricians and paediatricians also remain divided over whether

TABLE II — *Effect of corticosteroids given prior to preterm delivery on risk of early neonatal death*

Study	Experiment n	(%)	Control n	(%)	Odds ratio (95% CI)	Graph of odds ratios and confidence intervals
Liggins GC et al (1972)	36/532	(6·77)	60/538	(11·15)	0·58 (0·38–0·89)	
Block MF et al (1977)	1/69	(1·45)	5/61	(8·20)	0·22 (0·04–1·12)	
Schutte MF et al (1979)	3/64	(4·69)	12/58	(20·69)	(0·23) (0·08–0·67)	
Taeusch HW Jr et al (1979)	5/56	(8·93)	7/71	(9·86)	0·90 (0·27–2·96)	
Doran TA et al (1980)	2/81	(2·47)	10/63	(15·87)	0·18 (0·05–0·57)	
Teramo K et al (1980)	0/38	(0·00)	0/47	(0·00)	1·00 (1·00–1·00)	
Gamsu HR et al (1989)	14/131	(10·69)	20/137	(14·60)	0·70 (0·34–1·44)	
Collaborative (1981)	36/371	(9·70)	37/372	(9·95)	0·97 (0·60–1·58)	
Morales WJ et al (1986)	7/121	(5·79)	13/124	(10·48)	0·54 (0·22–1·33)	
Papageorgiou AN et al (1979)	1/71	(1·41)	5/75	(6·67)	0·27 (0·05–1·36)	
Morrison JC et al (1978)	2/67	(2·99)	7/59	(11·86)	0·26 (0·07–1·03)	
Schmidt PL et al (1984)	5/34	(14·71)	5/31	(16·13)	0·90 (0·24–3·42)	
Typical odds ratio (95% Confidence interval)					0·59 (0·47–0·75)	

131

administration of corticosteroids to a woman expected to deliver preterm reduces her baby's risk of dying. This divided opinion reflects uncertainties that have resulted from type II errors. Table II displays data derived from the 12 controlled trials reporting mortality data.[32] It shows that, for all of the trials, estimates of the effect of antenatal corticosteroids are consistent with the hypothesis that these drugs reduce the risk of early neonatal death. In terms of statistical significance, however, in only three of the 12 trials can chance be rejected as a likely explanation for the reduction observed. Arraying and synthesising all of the available data in a meta-analysis in this way expose the type II errors that seem likely to have been made in most of the trials.

GUIDING CLINICAL RESEARCH

In addition to clarifying options for clinical practice, the results of meta-analyses are helpful (if not essential) for clarifying the questions that should be addressed in clinical research. Firstly, meta-analyses may suggest completely new hypotheses. For example, a meta-analysis of the results of four controlled trials of continuous electronic intrapartum fetal heart monitoring yielded an hypothesis which had not emerged from less systematic reviews of the available evidence.[33] The meta-analysis suggested that babies whose heart rate had been monitored continuously, and whose acid-base status had been assessed when worrying traces had been observed, were less likely to experience seizures within 48 hours of birth than babies whose heart rate had been monitored using intermittent auscultation. This meta-analysis influenced the design of a further, very large clinical experiment, the results of which confirmed the validity of the hypothesis that had been generated by the meta-analysis.[34][35]

Secondly, meta-analyses can be used to test existing hypotheses. For example, extrapolation from the results of animal studies and underpowered trials in humans led to the hypothesis that fibrinolytic treatment was ineffective if started more than six hours after the onset of pain heralding an acute myocardial infarction. The results of a meta-analysis of the relevant randomised trials suggested that this view might be mistaken,[36] and these observations promoted sufficient uncertainty about the validity of prevailing wisdom that substantial numbers of the relevant patients were subsequently recruited to a very large trial of fibrinolysis. The results of this trial led to confident rejection of the hypothesis that fibrinolysis must be started less than six hours after the onset of pain for its beneficial effects to be manifested.[37]

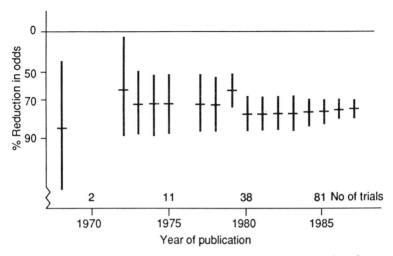

Cumulative estimates of the extent to which prophylactic antibiotics reduce the odds of serious postoperative infection after caesarean section[39]

Finally, meta-analyses may indicate that some questions about the effects of care have already been answered with considerable confidence, and that further research is inappropriate.[38] As can be seen from the data shown in the figure, for example, strong evidence has been available for two decades that the risk of serious postoperative infection can be reduced by routine antibiotic prophylaxis at the time of caesarean section.[39] Had this evidence been presented to obstetricians, clinical researchers, and women themselves 15 years ago, a policy of prophylaxis might have been adopted more widely in clinical practice, and researchers and women might have questioned the need for the many placebo controlled trials conducted after that time. As it is, women continue to be invited to participate in studies of antibiotic prophylaxis at caesarean section using placebo controls.

Improvements in the quality of reviews of clinical research

Well conducted meta-analyses are, to use Haynes' helpful terminology, examples of 'advanced clinical research'.[40] They can epitomise the kind of methodologically sound review article called for by Kass,[5] Mulrow,[11] and Oxman and Guyatt.[15] If appropriate steps are taken to reduce biases in the selection and analysis of data in meta-

133

analyses,[12] [14] there will be an improvement in the quality of evidence available for guiding clinical practice and research.

It is probably partly because these more formal, quantitative reviews have been judged to meet the needs both of clinicians and of clinical scientists so effectively that the numbers of meta-analyses appearing in biomedical journals have grown so rapidly.[12] [41] [42] Published reports of meta-analyses began to increase in frequency in the early 1980s. For the years prior to 1982, a MEDLINE search could be expected to yield an average of about one meta-analysis a year; between 1982 and 1985 the average annual yield was about 15.[42] Since 1986, the number of meta-analyses listed by MEDLINE has more than doubled every year, and a MEDLINE search using the MeSH term META-ANALYSIS and the text word 'meta-analysis' yielded 231 citations for 1989 (Dickersin, personal communication).

Most of the meta-analyses published in biomedical journals have been 'stand alone reviews'. These meta-analyses have usually focused either on a specific disease, such as breast cancer,[43] [44] or on a specific form of intervention, such as antiplatelet agents.[45] In addition, collections of meta-analyses relating to the treatment of duodenal ulcer[46] and care during pregnancy and childbirth[47] have been published in books.

Quite apart from their role as a way of improving the quality of 'stand alone' review articles, however, meta-analyses have an important part to play in helping to set new evidence in proper context. Reports of primary research should begin by referring, in the Introduction, to the results of a systematically conducted, published review of the results of relevant previously reported studies, explaining why the current study was justified. The Discussion section of the report should set the data generated by the new study in the context of all the evidence available at the time of analysis.

An exemplary presentation of new evidence is provided by the report of the first study in the series of international studies of infarct survival (ISIS).[48] ISIS 1 was designed to provide a statistically powerful test of the hypothesis that β blockade after myocardial infarction reduces the risk of early mortality. The Introduction to the report explained that this hypothesis had already received support from a meta-analysis of the results of all previously reported similar trials.[49] After the Materials and Methods and the Results of the new study had been presented, the Discussion section of the paper was used to integrate the results of the newly reported study with the available results of all other randomised trials of β blockade after myocardial infarction. Thus the authors based their inferences on a systematically conducted analysis incorporating all the relevant data that they had been able to obtain.

If meta-analysis becomes more widely used in reports of new evidence in this way, this will certainly place some journal editors in difficulties. A *Lancet* editorial referred to the meta-analysis presented in the Discussion section of the 10 page report of the ISIS 1 trial as a 'lengthy tailpiece', and, though acknowledging that 'there is a good case for such analyses', went on to state 'if anyone suggests that they should become a regular feature of clinical trial reports the *Lancet* will lead the opposition'.[50]

A dilemma undoubtedly faces editors of printed journals who wish to reconcile space constraints with the need to increase the scientific quality of reviews, whether these are of the 'stand alone' variety or components of reports of original research. This dilemma results not only from the fact that formal reviews may tend to take up more space than the kind of informal review that has been usual in the past, but also because substantial duplication of previously published information will be required if meta-analyses are to be updated efficiently as new evidence becomes available.

These problems are not insuperable. They can be addressed successfully by arranging for meta-analyses to be updated continuously within electronic management systems as new evidence becomes available, and then using these systems as the source of both printed and electronic publications.[51]

One example of a systematic, continuously updated review: evidence about the effects of care during pregnancy and childbirth

In 1976 a plan was outlined for reviewing evidence about the effects of perinatal care, applying the principles outlined above. The plan involved: first identifying as high a proportion as possible of properly controlled trials of perinatal care; then synthesising the results of similar trials in meta-analyses to reduce random error; and finally making arrangements for updating these analyses continuously as new data became available.

Because of concern about underascertainment of relevant studies,[18][52] a hand search of 60 'core' journals, beginning with the volumes published in 1950, was initiated in addition to conducting MEDLINE searches of reports published since 1966.[53][54] So far,

135

over 5000 reports of perinatal trials published in more than 250 journals have been identified and classified. In addition, details of unpublished perinatal trials were sought by surveying 42 000 obstetricians and paediatricians in the 18 countries in which the vast majority of controlled trials in perinatal medicine have been conducted.[55] This was done in an attempt to address the problems presented by publication bias and its potentially adverse effect on the validity of reviews.[56]

As trials were identified in these ways, details about each of them were entered into an electronic management system. This system has been the starting point for commissioning systematic reviews covering most elements of perinatal care. Reviewers who have agreed to collaborate in the project have been provided with listings of trials likely to be relevant to their areas of responsibility, and given guidelines for assessing the methodological quality of these studies, and for abstracting the results in a form suitable for presentation in meta-analyses.[18] These meta-analyses have been held in electronic form within the management system. When the results of only one trial are available to assess the effects of a particular form of care, these are incorporated in the system despite the fact that this does not, as such, represent a meta-analysis. For this reason the analyses within the system are referred to as 'overviews'.

More than 400 overviews of perinatal trials (largely concerned with obstetric care) have been published so far. Although some of these analyses have been published as articles in clinical journals,[32] [57–63] the most comprehensive collection has been published in a 1500 page, two volume book,[47] the principal conclusions of which are also available in a 400 page paperback summary.[64] Both books end with four appendices listing forms of care that have been shown to reduce the risk of negative outcomes; forms of care that appear to be promising but require further evaluation; forms of care with unknown effects; and forms of care that are so unlikely to have beneficial effects that they should be abandoned. These appendices thus summarise evidence of relevance not only for clinical practice, but also for deciding clinical research priorities. A sequel to this formal review of the effects of obstetric and midwifery care, reviewing the effects of neonatal paediatric care, is in press.[65]

The registers of published and unpublished randomised trials contained within the management system are being updated on a continuing basis. As the results of new trials become available, they are being reviewed by one of about 30 'overview editors' (almost all of whom are also authors of chapters in the book) and then, if appropriate, incorporated in existing or new overviews held in the management system. As recommended by Mulrow *et al*,[20] structured commentaries exist for an increasing proportion of these analyses, and these are being used to make preparations for efficient publication of second editions of the books (probably on compact disk as well as on paper) in about five years' time.

During the interval between printed editions of the books, the updated overviews and their structured commentaries are being downloaded from the master database every six months, and then distributed on floppy disks as an electronic journal.[66] A brief newsletter, drawing attention to some of the most important conclusions resulting from updating the overviews during the previous six months, is now also being published with each disk issue.

Incorporating new evidence in existing meta-analyses may result in previously tentative conclusions being sufficiently strengthened that the results of the updated meta-analyses should be used as a basis for guiding clinical practice. For example, evidence derived from six trials of prophylactic administration of surfactant in newborn infants was presented in meta-analyses published in the book.[67] Within six months of the book going to press, data from a further five randomised trials of prophylactic surfactant had become available. Incorporation of this new evidence in the meta-analyses confirmed beyond reasonable doubt that prophylactic surfactant administration results in a substantial reduction in neonatal morbidity and mortality.[68] [69]

On other occasions, the strengthened conclusion derived from an updated meta-analysis will be that a form of care in widespread use should be called into serious question. For example, evidence published in the book, which was derived from three controlled trials, suggested that a very common obstetric practice—using oxytocic drugs when there has been prelabour rupture of membranes at term—might be doing more harm than good.[70] Incorporating the results of two additional trials in the meta-analysis after the book had gone to press strengthened this view, and this confirmatory analysis was published in electronic form just six months after the publication of the book.[71] The editorial commentary suggested that if this questionable form of care was to be offered to women at all, it should only be in the context of properly controlled trials to assess its effects systematically.

Even if the results of an updated meta-analysis have no immediate implications for changing the direction of either clinical practice or research, it may still be helpful to make them available efficiently to confirm previous recommendations. This can be illustrated using the meta-analysis of trials of low dose aspirin given to women at statistically increased risk of developing proteinuric pre-eclampsia. The version of the meta-analysis published in the book (table IIIa) presented results from two controlled trials, both of which suggested that the incidence of proteinuric pre-eclampsia might be reduced by this antiplatelet agent.[72] The authors concluded that, although encouraging, these results had no immediate implications for clinical practice because no beneficial impact on substantive adverse outcomes of pregnancy (mortality or serious morbidity) had been shown. Much larger trials were required to assess whether administering low dose aspirin could have beneficial effects in these terms. The results of an updated version of the meta-analysis, now incorporating the results of seven trials, and disseminated six months after the book was published (table IIIb), confirmed the continuing validity of the earlier recommendations. The updated version of this particular meta-analysis illustrates another advantage of electronic publishing: one of the trials originally included in the analysis was later excluded when it became known to the overview editor that the allocation of participants to the two experimental groups had not been truly random and so may have been biased.

The presentation of this meta-analysis also illustrates how electronic publication might help to speed up the process of generating new evidence. The editorial commentary invited anyone interested in helping to assess the effects of aspirin on mortality and serious morbidity to collaborate in a multicentre trial which is seeking additional collaborators.[73] Details of the trial, including the address and telephone number of the co-ordinating centre, are accessible within the same electronic publication as the meta-analysis.[74]

Finally, it has been encouraging to observe that aspects of practice for which no properly controlled trials were available at the time the book went to press (augmentation for poor progress in labour and administration of magnesium sulphate for tocolysis are examples) have been the subject of investigations published subsequently. During the year after publication of the book, the results of these studies have formed the basis for establishing new meta-analyses, which have then been published electronically.

Although a working system now exists through which meta-analyses of controlled trials of perinatal care can be updated and created as new evidence becomes available, considerable scope exists

TABLE IIIa — *Effect of low dose aspirin on incidence of proteinuric pre-eclampsia: evidence published in print, August 1989*[72]

| Study | Experiment | | Control | | Odds ratio (95% CI) | Graph of odds ratios and confidence intervals |
	n	(%)	n	(%)		0·01 0·1 0·5 1 2 10 100
Wallenberg HCS et al (1986)	0/23	(0·00)	8/23	(34·78)	0·09 (0·02–0·42)	
Beaufils M et al (1984)	0/48	(0·00)	6/45	(13·33)	0·11 (0·02–0·58)	
Typical odds ratio (95% Confidence interval)					0·10 (0·03–0·31)	

TABLE IIIb — *Effects of low dose aspirin in incidence of proteinuric pre-eclampsia: evidence published electronically, February 1990*[73]

Study	Experiment n	Experiment (%)	Control n	Control (%)	Odds ratio (95% CI)	Graph of odds ratios and confidence intervals
Wallenburg HCS et al (1986)	0/23	(0·00)	8/23	(34·78)	0·09 (0·02–0·42)	
Schiff E et al (1989)	1/34	(2·94)	7/31	(22·58)	0·17 (0·04–0·73)	
Sibai BM et al (1989)	0/30	(0·00)	0/10	(0·00)	1·00 (1·00–1·00)	
McParland PJ et al (1989)	0/36	(0·00)	9/42	(21·43)	0·13 (0·03–0·50)	
Breart G (unpublished)	5/156	(3·21)	8/73	(10·96)	0·24 (0·07–0·78)	
Benigni A et al (1989)	0/17	(0·00)	0/16	(0·00)	1·00 (1·00–1·00)	
Railton AS et al (1988)	4/29	(13·79)	4/14	(28·57)	0·39 (0·08–1·95)	
Typical odds ratio (95% Confidence interval)					0·18 (0·09–0·33)	

for improving the validity and efficiency of this process. Predictably, the availability of resources is one of the constraints preventing these improvements; but there is reason to hope that useful progress can be made nevertheless. Members of the editorial team managing and developing the system are continuing to learn, by trial and error, how to improve it. Hopefully their experience and that of others working along similar lines will be helpful to others who are interested in assembling and synthesising information in a similar way for other aspects of health care.

Conclusions

It is surely a great criticism of our profession that we have not organised a critical summary, by specialty or subspecialty, adapted periodically, of all relevant randomised controlled trials.

Archie Cochrane, 1979[75]

Until recently, clinical investigators have usually failed to apply scientific principles to the process of reviewing evidence derived from clinical research. As a result, patients have been denied effective forms of care; they have been offered ineffective and hazardous forms of care; and they have been involved in misconceived clinical research. If these problems are to be reduced, those reviewing evidence will have to take steps to minimise the various biases that can attend the review process, and use methods (like meta-analysis) to obtain estimates of association which are as precise as possible. Meta-analysis is required not only for 'stand alone' review articles, but also to set new evidence in proper context in the Discussion sections of reports of new research.

Wider adoption and application of scientific principles in these situations may pose editors of printed journals with a dilemma because systematic reviews of evidence tend to use more page space than traditional forms of review, particularly if they begin to replace the traditional form of discursive Discussion in reports of new research. In addition, editors may be reluctant to publish updated meta-analyses every time relevant new evidence is generated. These problems can be addressed by establishing electronic management systems facilitating continuous updating of meta-analyses, from which both paper and electronic publications can be produced when required.

Such electronic management systems already exist for meta-analyses of controlled trials in a number of topics, including

141

treatments for early breast cancer, anti-platelet agents, and perinatal care. There is no reason why the approach should not be extended to cover all clinical specialties. Although resources will be required if these developments are to be fostered efficiently, the order of support required would constitute a trivial fraction of the funds currently allocated for clinical and health services research, let alone the sums now spent on health care itself. The main requirement is not for resources, however. A more urgent need is wider acknowledgement that applying scientific principles to the review process should help to improve the quality of clinical and policy decisions, both about health care and about clinical research.

Acknowledgements

The work described in the penultimate section of this chapter has entailed collaboration with literally hundreds of people. Most of them have been acknowledged by name in *Effective Care in Pregnancy and Childbirth*; I reiterate my indebtedness to all of them here, and acknowledge my particular debts to Murray and Eleanor Enkin, Marc Keirse, Jini Hetherington, Sally Hunt, Mary Tinker, and Mark Starr. The main sources of funds for the work have been the Department of Health (London), the World Health Organisation, and Oxford University Press. I acknowledge with gratitude the helpful criticisms of earlier drafts of this paper provided by Tom Chalmers, Kay Dickersin, Brian Haynes, David Paintin, Richard Peto, Ken Warren, Elizabeth Wilson, and my colleagues at the National Perinatal Epidemiology Unit. Finally, I acknowledge my debt to Archie Cochrane, who first showed me how to reduce bias in treatment comparisons, and thus provided me with a compass to help me find my way through the dense jungle of clinical research publications.

1 Cited in: Leitch I. The collection and dissemination of information on nutrition with special reference to the United Kingdom. *Prog Food Nutr Sci* 1976:2:59.
2 Light RJ, Pillemer DB. *Summing up: the science of reviewing research*. Cambridge, Massachusetts: Harvard University Press, 1984.
3 Pillemer DB. Conceptual issues in research synthesis. *Journal of Special Education* 1984;**18**:27–40.
4 Jackson GB. Methods for integrative reviews. *Review of Educational Research* 1980;**50**:438–60.
5 Kass EH. Reviewing reviews. In: Warren KS, ed. *Coping with the biomedical literature*. New York: Praeger, 1981:79–91.
6 Cooper HM. Scientific guidelines for conducting integrative research reviews. *Review of Educational Research* 1982:52:291–302.

7 Cooper HM. *The integrative research review*. Beverly Hills, California: Sage Publications, 1984.
8 Einarson TR, McGhan WF, Bootman JL, Sabers DL. Meta-analysis: quantitative integration of independent research results. *Am J Hosp Pharm* 1985;**42**:1957–64.
9 Morgan PP. Review articles: 2. The literature jungle. *Can Med Assoc J* 1986;**134**:98–9.
10 Huth EJ. Needed: review articles with more scientific rigour. *Ann Intern Med* 1987;**106**:470–1.
11 Mulrow CD. The medical review article: state of the science. *Ann Intern Med* 1987;**104**:485–8.
12 Sacks HS, Berrier J, Reitman D, Ancona-Berk VA, Chalmers TC. Meta-analyses of randomized controlled trials. *N Engl J Med* 1987;**316**:450–5.
13 Collins R, Gray R, Godwin J, Peto R. Avoidance of large biases in the assessment of moderate treatment effects: the need for systematic overviews. *Stat Med* 1987;**6**:245–250.
14 L'Abbé KA, Detsky AS, O'Rourke K. Meta-analysis in clinical research. *Ann Intern Med* 1987;**107**:224–32.
15 Oxman AD, Guyatt GH. Guidelines for reading literature reviews. *Can Med Assoc J* 1988;**138**:697–703.
16 Thacker SB. Meta-analysis: a quantitative approach to research integration. *JAMA* 1988;**259**:1685–9.
17 Ellenberg SS. Meta-analysis: the quantitative approach to research review. *Semin Oncol* 1988;**15**:472–81.
18 Chalmers I, Hetherington J, Elbourne D, Keirse MJNC, Enkin M. Materials and methods used in synthesizing evidence to evaluate the effects of care during pregnancy and childbirth. In: Chalmers I, Enkin M, Keirse MJNC, eds. *Effective care in pregnancy and childbirth*. Oxford: Oxford University Press, 1989:39–65.
19 Williamson JW, German PS, Weiss R, Skinner EA, Bowes F. Health science information management and continuing education of physicians. *Ann Intern Med* 1989;**110**:151–60.
20 Mulrow CD, Thacker SB, Pugh JA. A proposal for more informative abstracts of review articles. *Ann Intern Med* 1988;**108**:613–5.
21 Wolf FM. *Meta-analysis: quantitative methods for research synthesis*. London: Sage Publications, 1986.
22 Cooper HM, Rosenthal R. Statistical versus traditional procedures for summarising research findings. *Psychol Bull* 1980;**87**:442–9.
23 Hedges LV. Commentary. *Stat Med* 1987;**6**:381–5.
24 Jones LV, Fiske DW. Models for testing the significance of combined results. *Psychol Bull* 1953;**50**:375–82.
25 Mosteller FM, Bush RR. Selected quantitative techniques. In: Lindsay G, ed. *Handbook of social psychology*: Vol 1. *Theory and method*. Cambridge, Mass: Addison-Wesley, 1954:289–334.
26 Beecher HK. The powerful placebo. *JAMA* 1955;**159**:1602–6.
27 Light RJ, Smith PV. Accumulating evidence: procedures for resolving contradictions among different research studies. *Harvard Educational Review* 1971;**41**:429–71.
28 Glass GV. Primary, secondary and meta-analysis of research. *Educational Research* 1976:**5**:3–8.
29 Longnecker MP, Berlin JA, Orza MJ, Chalmers TC. A meta-analysis of alcohol consumption in relation to breast cancer. *JAMA* 1988;**260**:652–6.
30 Peto R. Why do we need systematic overviews of randomized trials? *Stat Med* 1987;**6**:233–40.
31 Roberton NRC. Advances in respiratory distress syndrome. *Br Med J* 1982;**284**:917–8.
32 Crowley P, Chalmers I, Keirse MJNC. The effects of corticosteroid adminis-

tration before preterm delivery: an overview of the evidence from controlled trials. *Br J Obstet Gynaecol* 1990;**97**:11–25.

33 Chalmers I. Randomised trials of fetal monitoring 1973–1977. In: Thalhammer O, Baumgarten K, Pollak A, eds. *Perinatal medicine*. Stuttgart: Georg Thieme, 1979:260–5.

34 MacDonald D, Grant A, Sheridan-Pereira M, Boylan P, Chalmers I. The Dublin randomized controlled trial of intrapartum fetal heart rate monitoring. *Am J Obstet Gynecol* 1985;**152**:524–39.

35 Grant A, O'Brien N, Joy M, Hennessy E, MacDonald D. Cerebral palsy among children born in the Dublin randomized trial of intrapartum monitoring. *Lancet* 1989;ii:1233–6.

36 Yusuf S, Peto R, Lewis T, Collins R, Sleight P. Beta blockade during and after myocardial infarction: an overview of the randomised trials. *Prog Cardiovasc Dis* 1985;**XXVII** (5):336–71.

37 ISIS-2 Collaborative Group. Randomised trial of intravenous streptokinase, oral aspirin, both, or neither among 17,187 cases of suspected acute myocardial infarction: ISIS-2. *Lancet* 1988;ii:349–60.

38 Baum ML, Anish DS, Chalmers TC, Sacks HS, Smith H, Fagerstrom RM. A survey of clinical trials of antibiotic prophylaxis in colon surgery: evidence against further use of no-treatment controls. *N Engl J Med* 1981;**305**:795–9.

39 Enkin M, Enkin E, Chalmers I, Hemminki E. Prophylactic antibiotics in association with caesarean section. In: Chalmers I, Enkin M, Keirse MJNC, eds. *Effective care in pregnancy and childbirth*. Oxford: Oxford University Press, 1989:1246–69.

40 Haynes RB. Loose connections between peer-reviewed clinical journals and clinical practice. *Ann Intern Med* 1990;**113**:724–8.

41 Halvorsen KT. Combining results from independent investigations: meta-analysis in medical research. In: Bailar J, Mosteller F, eds. *Medical uses of statistics*. Boston: NEJM Books, 1986:392–416.

42 Dickersin K, Higgins K, Meinert CL. Identification of meta-analyses: the need for standard terminology. *Controlled Clin Trials* 1990;**11**:52–66.

43 Early Breast Cancer Trialists' Collaborative Group. Effects of adjuvant tamoxifen and of cytotoxic therapy on mortality in early breast cancer: and overview of 62 randomized trials among 28,896 women. *N Engl J Med* 1988;**319**:1681–92.

44 Early Breast Cancer Trialists' Collaborative Group. *Treatment of early breast cancer*. Volume 1. *Worldwide evidence 1985–1990*. Oxford: Oxford University Press, 1990.

45 Antiplatelet Trialists' Collaboration. Secondary prevention of vascular disease by prolonged antiplatelet treatment. *Br Med J*. 1988;**296**:320–31.

46 Poynard T, Pignon JP. *Acute treatment of duodenal ulcer: analysis of 293 randomized clinical trials*. London: John Libbey, 1989.

47 Chalmers I, Enkin M, Keirse MJNC, eds. *Effective care in pregnancy and childbirth*. Oxford: Oxford University Press, 1989.

48 ISIS-1 Collaborative Group. Randomised trial of intravenous atenolol among 16,027 cases of suspected acute myocardial infarction: ISIS-1. *Lancet* 1986;ii:57–66.

49 Yusuf S, Collins R, Peto R, Furberg C, Stampfer MJ, Goldhaber SZ, *et al.* Intravenous and intracoronary fibrinolytic therapy in acute myocardial infarction: overview of results on mortality, reinfarction and side effects from 33 randomized controlled trials. *Eur Heart J* 1985;**6**:556–85.

50 Anonymous Intravenous β-blockade during acute myocardial infarction. *Lancet* 1986;ii:79–80.

51 Chalmers I. Electronic publications for updating controlled trial reviews. *Lancet* 1986;ii:287.

52 Dickersin K, Hewitt P, Mutch L, Chalmers I, Chalmers TC. Perusing the literature. Comparison of MEDLINE searching with a perinatal trials database. *Controlled Clin Trials* 1985;**6**:306–17.

53 National Perinatal Epidemiology Unit. *A classified bibliography of controlled trials in perinatal medicine, 1940–1984.* Oxford: Oxford University Press, 1985.

54 Chalmers I, Hetherington J, Newdick M, Mutch L, Grant A, Enkin M, *et al.* The Oxford database of perinatal trials: developing a register of published reports of controlled trials. *Controlled Clin Trials* 1986;7:306–25.

55 Hetherington J, Chalmers I, Dickersin K, Meinert C. Retrospective and prospective identification of controlled trials: lessons from a survey of obstetricians and paediatricians. *Pediatrics* 1989;84:374–80.

56 Dickersin K. The existence of publication bias and risk factors for its occurrence. *JAMA* 1990;263:1385–9.

57 Collins R, Yusuf S, Peto R. Overview of randomised trials of diuretics in pregnancy. *Br Med J* 1985;290:17–23.

58 King JF, Grant A, Keirse MJNC, Chalmers I. Beta-mimetics in preterm labour: an overview of the randomized controlled trials. *Br J Obstet Gynaecol* 1988;95:211–22.

59 Prendiville W, Elbourne D, Chalmers I. The effects of routine oxytocic administration in the management of the third stage of labour: an overview of the evidence from controlled trials. *Br J Obstet Gynaecol* 1988;95:3–16.

60 Elbourne D, Prendiville W, Chalmers I. Choice of oxytocic preparation for routine use in the management of the third stage of labour: an overview of the evidence from controlled trials. *Br J Obstet Gynaecol* 1988;95:17–30.

61 Grant A. The choice of suture materials and techniques for repair of perineal trauma: an overview of the evidence from controlled trials. *Br J Obstet Gynaecol* 1989;96:1281–9.

62 Goldstein P, Berrier J, Rosen S, Sacks HC, Chalmers TC. A meta-analysis of randomized control trials of progestational agents in pregnancy. *Br J Obstet Gynaecol* 1989;96:265–7.

63 Keirse MJNC. Progestogen administration in pregnancy may prevent preterm delivery. *Br J Obstet Gynaecol* 1990;97:149–54.

64 Enkin M, Keirse MJNC, Chalmers I. *A guide to effective care during pregnancy and childbirth.* Oxford: Oxford University Press, 1989.

65 Sinclair JC, Bracken M, eds. *Effective care of the newborn infant.* Oxford: Oxford University Press. (In press).

66 Chalmers I, ed. *The Oxford database of perinatal trials.* Version 1.2, Disk Issue 6. Oxford: Oxford University Press, Autumn 1991.

67 Tyson J, Silverman W, Reisch J. Immediate care of the newborn infant. In: Chalmers I, Enkin M, Keirse MJNC, eds. *Effective care in pregnancy and childbirth.* Oxford: Oxford University Press, 1989:1293–312.

68 Soll RF. Prophylactic administration of natural surfactant extract. In: Chalmers I, ed. *Oxford database of perinatal trials.* Version 1.1, Disk Issue 3. Oxford: Oxford University Press, February 1990:5207.

69 Soll RF. Prophylactic administration of synthetic surfactant extract. In: Chalmers I, ed. *Oxford database of perinatal trials.* Version 1.1, Disk Issue 3. Oxford: Oxford University Press, February 1990:5253.

70 Grant J, Keirse MJNC. Prelabour rupture of the membranes at term. In: Chalmers I, Enkin M, Keirse MJNC, eds. *Effective care in pregnancy and childbirth.* Oxford: Oxford University Press, 1989:1112–7.

71 Keirse MJNC. Active management of prelabour rupture of membranes at term. In: Chalmers I, ed. *Oxford database of perinatal trials.* Version 1.1, Disk Issue 3. Oxford: Oxford University Press, February 1990:3272.

72 Collins R, Wallenburg HCS. Pharmacological prevention and treatment of hypertensive disorders in pregnancy. In: Chalmers I, Enkin M, Keirse MJNC, eds. *Effective care in pregnancy and childbirth.* Oxford: Oxford University Press, 1989:512–33.

73 Collins R. Anti-platelet administration for prophylaxis and treatment of pre-eclampsia and IUGR. In: Chalmers I, ed. *Oxford database of perinatal trials.* Version 1.1, Disk Issue 3. February 1990:4000.

74 Farrell B. MRC Collaborative Low dose Aspirin Studies in Pregnancy (CLASP). In: Chalmers I, ed. *Oxford database of perinatal trials.* Version 1.1, Disk Issue 3. Oxford: Oxford University Press, February 1990:4190.
75 Cochrane AL. 1931–1971: a critical review, with particular reference to the medical profession. In: *Medicines for the year 2000.* London: Office of Health Economics, 1979.

PART 4
THE TECHNOLOGIES OF INFORMATION

From papyrus to parchment to paper to pixels: information technology and the future of biomedical publishing

KENNETH S WARREN

We remain immured in ways of thinking about and handling information that were developed centuries and millennia ago. The record of the written word begins with virtually indestructible clay tablets, such as those found in the library of the Assyrian king Assurbanipal at Nineveh (seventh century BC), which contained documents on history, mythology, agriculture, medicine, and mathematics.

Papyrus

It is generally believed that libraries, which contained perishable papyrus scrolls, began in Egypt. The first of consequence was a temple built by Rameses II of Egypt in the thirteenth century BC, which contained sacred literature. The entrance bore the inscription 'Medicine for the Soul.' The scrolls, which consisted of papyrus sheets glued together, were commonly called biblion, derived from Byblos, the port from which papyrus was shipped to the Mediterranean world. The most famous library of the ancient world was founded by the Ptolemies, Greek rulers of Egypt, about 300 BC in Alexandria, and contained about 600 000 papyrus scrolls. It was, unfortunately, destroyed by fire in the early Christian era, leading to such a sense of loss that libraries ever since have striven to

149

preserve virtually everything, presumably forever (see Stanislaw Lem below).

Parchment

The second of the great ancient Greek libraries was in the city of Pergamum in western Turkey. Because the supply of papyrus from Egypt was uncertain, parchment, made from the skin of sheep or goats, was used instead. This made possible the codex, or book, in the form we know today. As parchment, unlike papyrus, does not crack when folded, it can be sewn easily and can be written on on both sides. The library of Pergamum contained about 200 000 such volumes.

Parchment continued to be used throughout the Middle Ages, largely in the scriptoria of monasteries, which, though low on quantity, were capable of producing magnificently illuminated volumes in bejeweled leather bindings. In the thirteenth century universities began to rival monasteries in their demand for books; by the early fourteenth century the library of the Sorbonne contained close to 2000 volumes. During this period paper began to replace parchment.

Paper and printing

Paper, made largely of bamboo fibres, appeared in China sometime around AD 100. Arabs acquired the art of paper making when they captured the central Asian city of Samarkand from the Chinese in the eighth century AD. Paper mills were soon established in the Arab world, including one in Baghdad which used linen rags as raw material. The use of paper spread throughout north Africa and thence to Moorish Spain. Paper making became widespread throughout Europe by the fourteenth century. Rag paper continued to be used until the middle of the nineteenth century when it was superceded by papers based on acidic wood pulp. It is worthy of note that many books printed on acidic paper from the late nineteenth century onwards are deteriorating and can be saved only by inefficient and expensive deacidification processes.

Although a form of movable type for printing had been invented as early as the eleventh century AD in China, its use had not spread beyond that country's borders. In the mid-fifteenth century the modern method of printing, using movable and reusable type, was founded by Gutenberg and his associates. The combination of paper and movable type made possible a veritable explosion in output of printed documents. Scholars have located some 40 000 editions, averaging about 200 copies each, printed in the 50 year period from Gutenberg's invention to the turn of the century. Thus, in a mere half century, more copies of books were printed than had been copied throughout several preceding centuries.

In 1961, just prior to the next great advance in technology, Derek de Solla Price stated laconically, 'Roughly speaking, both the world population of book titles and the sizes of all the great libraries double in about 20 years. If we allow that in some 500 years of book production there must have been some twenty five doubling periods, this will give about 30 000 000 books alive today, a figure conforming well with normal estimates.'[1]

In addition to the evolution and growth of book production and the libraries which store them, the particularly important role of journals in the development of science must be considered in the present context. This matter was graphically depicted by de Solla Price in his book *Science Since Babylon* (fig 1). The scientific journal and the device of the 'learned paper' were invented in the seventeenth century. The earliest surviving journal is the *Philosophical Transactions of the Royal Society of London* (founded in 1665), followed by several similar publications by other national academies in Europe. Again we see a geometric progression with about 100 journals at the beginning of the nineteenth century, 1000 by its middle, and 10 000 at its termination. Figure 1, which continues this remarkable growth through the twentieth century, led de Solla Price to claim that 'it became evident by about 1830 that the process had reached a point of absurdity: no scientist could read all the journals or keep sufficiently conversant with all published work that might be relevant to his interest.' This resulted in the rise of abstract journals and, in turn, their geometric growth. de Solla Price suggested that the time may have come for a new approach, beyond abstracts, for the compression of information.[1] Such an approach might necessitate a qualitative rather than a merely quantitative approach to information, a matter which will be discussed below.

Pixels

The latest stage in the evolution of the substrates on which information is displayed is the pixel, defined as the smallest element of an image that can be individually processed in a video display system. This term is derived from pix, the plural of pic or picture, plus el, or element. As this is the major means by which computerised material is displayed and as the computer is the primary

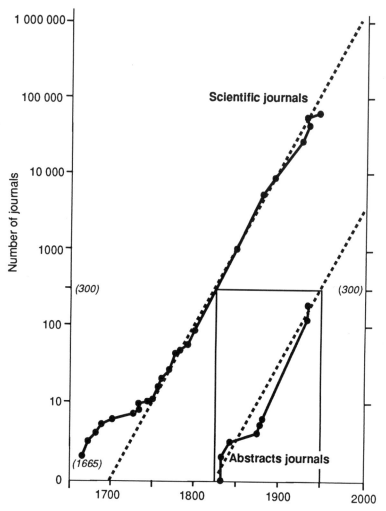

FIG 1—*Total number of scientific journals and abstract journals founded, as a function of date*[1]

instrument of the long impending information revolution, we are now in an age in which we are being bombarded simultaneously with information on paper and pixels.

The roots of the computer go back to the abacus, which was developed thousands of years ago. A major step in the evolution of a series of related instruments was the invention by the nineteenth century British mathematician Charles Babbage of an analytical

152

engine to carry out a wide range of calculating tasks. During the second world war the concept of the universal computer became established with John von Neumann's outline of the critical elements of a computer system. It was not until the middle 1970s that personal computers, which empower vast numbers of potential end users, began to be mass produced.

Jerome Rubin, physicist, lawyer, and developer of Lexis, recently wrote, 'Charles Babbage hailed the printing press as the great accelerator of progress—"Until printing was very generally spread," [Babbage claimed] "civilization scarcely advanced by slow and languid steps; since that art has become cheap its advances have become unparalleled, and its rate of progress vastly accelerated." Paradoxically, in developing his analytical engine, Babbage himself helped lay the foundation for the computer revolution transforming publishing—and our entire civilization—today.'[2] At the moment, however, the ability of the computer merely to facilitate production on paper— via computerised typesetting, laser printers, and desktop publishing software—adds a further dimension to the growth of scientific and medical information. Furthermore, output of essentially the same material can be produced simultaneously in many different forms (for example, full-fledged continuously updated texts, abbreviated versions for a variety of special interest groups, newsletters), and media (for example, paper, on line, compact discs, tapes, cards)

Inspired by these technological advances, the future of information systems has been described by science fiction writers and belleletrists. Stanislaw Lem wrote of an instrument called the Metainformationator which would 'extract from the dance of atoms only information that is genuine like mathematical theorems, fashion magazines, blueprints, historical chronicles, or a recipe for ion crumpets, or how to clean and iron a suit of asbestos, and poetry too, and scientific advice, and almanacs, and calendars, and secret documents, and anything that ever appeared in any newspaper in the universe, and telephone books of the future.'[3] Primo Levi described a pocket sized metal box called a Minibrain, a four track selector which could tell you 'how many women named Eleonora were operated on for appendicitis in Sicily in 1940, or how many of the suicides in the entire world from 1900 to date were both left handed and blond.'[4]

Medicine's failure to cope with information

The glut of information described above has had a disastrous effect on the ability of doctors to cope with information. After suffering in medical school from being stuffed with information, students frequently develop a syndrome known as 'cerveau gras' (CG); it is a state in which all desire to assimilate more information has been satiated. To prevent CG medical students have been begging for ways to circumvent the stuffing process. They desperately seek means by which they can efficiently obtain reliable information as needed. Therein lies the allure of the pixel.

Computer aided learning and knowledge systems remain inadequate, however, as do artificial intelligence based diagnostic and treatment systems, due to the time consuming task of developing them and keeping them up to date, the plethora of different hard and software systems used, and, as in the case of the artificial intelligence systems, their lack of precision, except when they are devoted to very narrow topics. In a recent article by Greenes and Shortliffe, two of the pioneers of medical informatics in the United States, it was stated that 'Despite years of research and development, computer based aids for diagnosis and treatment still remain largely curiosities and demonstration projects, rather than tools for routine use.'[5] The computer also serves as the major route of access to published reports through on-line and compact disc versions of MEDLINE, an information system which, while the best system available, is relatively inefficient and costly both in time and money, particularly in regard to clinical decision-making.

Furthermore, cognitive psychologists have shown that a large amount of knowledge is required to develop expertise in technical subjects such as language fluency, chess, or physics.[6] For each topic about 10 000 items must be entered into long term memory at a cost of 10 seconds each and must also be multiply indexed. It has therefore been estimated that it takes about 12 years to train an expert. Studies have also shown that expertise is relatively narrow— that is, though a medical student cannot cope with a cardiological problem like a cardiologist, neither can an endocrinologist.[7] Hope has been offered, however, that we may increasingly be able to use computers to supplement short term memory through pattern detection and long term memory by consulting expert systems.[6] Unfortunately that time has still not arrived.

Medical education

Harold Schoolman of the National Library of Medicine has recently written, 'for many years medical schools have abdicated any role in educating their students for the information age. If pressed, they would answer that it was the function of continuing medical education. Medical schools now recognise that their classical paradigm, in which medical students were to learn the knowledge base of medicine, cannot be achieved. The knowledge base is too large and is changing too rapidly. So in recent years we have been confronted with a series of reports advocating curricular revisions. These revisions recognise the fundamental role of the physician as a decision maker. To be an effective decision maker, one must be an efficient information processor.'[8] However, the most recent conference on this matter, *Medical Education: Time for Change*, ignored the role of information; it was not mentioned, even in passing, by any of the eminent speakers.[9]

Examples of medical school efforts to deal with the overwhelming information problem are Harvard's new pathway programme, McMaster's critical assessment teaching system, and Case Western Reserve's earlier course in information understanding and management. From its very inception Harvard's programme has put an emphasis on computer literacy as the answer to the problem. In the words of Dean Tosteson, 'Among the skills all doctors need, I would include both those required for learning and those essential for practicing medicine. The ability to use computers and other devices to manage information comfortably and efficiently will surely be required of all physicians in the coming decades. Greater attention to the use of these devices in the course of medical education would help current students to develop these learning skills.'[10] McMaster has focussed on critically appraising clinical reports, thereby enabling the student and the practising doctor to assess the validity and applicability of published evidence and to incorporate the results into patient management. 'It is based on the premise that to be effective in maintaining or improving the health of their patients clinicians must base the care they give on sound scientific evidence that it does more good than harm.'[11]

The Case Western Reserve University system was initiated in 1972 with a free subscription to the *New England Journal of Medicine* for all first and second year medical students and their teachers. The intent was to expose students to a quality journal with a broad range of articles, and to encourage teachers to cite articles in the journal.[12] This was associated with an elective course in biomedical and clinical information. The quantitative and qualitative aspects of the clinical and biomedical bodies of published reports were described, heuristics on how to deal with them presented (such as Franz Inglefinger's admonition to at least scan the *Lancet* or the *New*

England Journal of Medicine every week), and hands on exercises in retrieving information provided. Alas, the programme lapsed when those who initiated it left the university five years later.

Medical Education in the Information Age, the Association of American Medical Colleges' (AAMC) 1986 report on medical informatics, acknowledged 'the challenge for all physicians to organize and synthesize knowledge for clinical care in a manner that is efficient, efficacious and cost-effective.'[13] Though the AAMC advocated a central role for this relatively new discipline in medical education, a 1990 publication notes that, although a number of medical informatics departments were established in European medical schools in the past decade, the United States has developed only three, one of which is now defunct.[5] Another problem is that medical informatics itself places an overweening focus on machines and too little on understanding the complex system of information, its ecology, history, philosophy, and sociology. In the AAMC report informatics was described as being as 'like any other technology which is tool driven, the essential concepts and the discovery of new understanding coalesce about the subject matter because of the physical tool.'[14] Thus the publication emphasised the overwhelming role of the computer, for good or for ill (see below), in the future of information and medical education.

Medical practice

The Edinburgh Declaration of the World Conference on Medical Education in 1988 emphasised that 'continuity of learning throughout life' must be ensured.[15] The sad reality behind this statement is the failure of continuing medical education to maintain the knowledge base of practising doctors. In a critical appraisal of the efficacy of continuing medical education, 248 original articles on the subject were examined: only 32 were randomised trials, of which only seven met all pre-set criteria; only three of these assessed patient outcomes and only one showed any improvement.[16] In a more recent randomised trial of a continuing medical education course on hypertension for primary care doctors there was no lasting effect on doctor knowledge and no influence on lowering patients' blood pressure. The authors' conclusion was, 'Resources spent on institutional materials mailed to physicians may be wasted.'[17]

In a study by Covell *et al*[18] a questionnaire administered to 47 internists in California showed that doctors needed information on average once a week, and that they used print sources such as textbooks, journals, and drug information compendia more often than consultations. When the practices of these same individuals were observed by an interviewer, however, they generated about two questions for every three patients, about 70% of which were entirely unanswered; of the remaining 30%, other doctors and health professionals answered more than half and printed documents less than one fifth. The 'reasons print sources were not used included the age of textbooks in the office, poor organisation of journal articles, inadequate indexing of books and drug information sources, lack of knowledge of an appropriate source, and the time required to find the desired information.'[18]

A telephone survey of several hundred primary care practitioners and their opinion leaders throughout the USA by Williamson *et al* was devoted to the status of health science information management and continuing education.[19] When asked about their use of six recent clinical advances, such as glycated haemoglobin for diabetes control, 20% to 50% were not using or were not aware of such advances. Less than one third of the practitioners personally searched the literature when information was needed; two thirds claimed that the volume of published reports was unmanageable, and 90% of practitioners and opinion leaders evaluated the reports obtained on the basis of their own experience. All groups interviewed stated that summaries of recent articles and critical reviews were the most useful means of obtaining information. Over half of them said that telephone hotlines or expert networks would be very useful, and well under half claimed that obtaining complete articles from on line systems was sufficiently worthwhile. The conclusions of the authors were that 'physicians face a serious problem in their effort to keep current with recent medical advances. Science information management is a critical professional skill that is not adequately taught in undergraduate medical education. Too often practitioners "don't know what they don't know." '[19]

The Future of Information Systems for the Medical Sciences was the title of a 1987 Harris survey which included 98 basic science faculty members, 102 clinical faculty members, 99 medical students, 104 residents, 201 office based doctors, and 50 deans. Some of the relevant conclusions were that the information explosion has made computerised information systems essential, that medical students and professionals are still quite dependent on the printed word, and that office based doctors seem to be the least informed members of the medical community.[20]

The quantity/quality conundrum

Twenty three years ago, Margit Kraft, a renowned librarian, stated, 'The difference between a philosophy and a technique is that a philosophy sets goals, while a technique devises means to achieve these goals. If goals are nebulous, technique takes over and runs wild.'[21] Substitute technology for technique and computer for technology and it becomes clear that we are worshiping a machine in the hopes that it will solve a problem of immense scope and considerable complexity that has been with us for literally hundreds of years. First, we must view this problem historically; then, information must be seen as a dynamic, interactive system, for which mathematical models might be developed (even using the computer to do so) and verified by empirical studies. It is also essential that we focus on information qualitatively as well as quantitatively. Once we begin to understand the highly complex system we are dealing with, we may be able to devise approaches to make it more tractable and to use the computer as an instrument to fulfill our desires and needs.

As described at the beginning of this chapter, the successive development of papyrus, parchment, paper and printing, and the pixel based computer have each drastically increased the quantity of information (fig 1). This was facilitated not only by the remarkable growth of human populations but by the development of higher education and its output of a much greater proportion of producers of scientific and clinical information. In studies of scientific publications it was found that the ratios of papers to authors have remained constant over periods of 70 to 110 years, which suggests that the basic problem is a population rather than an information explosion.[22] The problem, however, has almost invariably been ascribed to the scientists' 'publish or perish' mentality, and many proposals have been made to limit their output of papers. One publication in the *New England Journal of Medicine*, more than a decade ago, proposed that no scientist should be allowed to publish more than five papers a year or 50 in a lifetime.[23]. This was countered by a recent article in the *New Scientist* that noted that such rules applied to the arts would have drastically curtailed the output of Mozart and Picasso.[24] In this context it is important to realise that an outstanding scientist is probably as rare as an outstanding composer, painter, or for that matter, football player.

An example of the pyramidal structure of excellence has recently been shown for basketball players (fig 2). It should be noted,

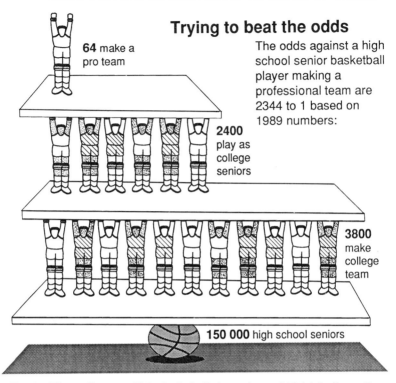

Trying to beat the odds

64 make a pro team

The odds against a high school senior basketball player making a professional team are 2344 to 1 based on 1989 numbers:

2400 play as college seniors

3800 make college team

150 000 high school seniors

FIG 2—*The quality pyramid for basketball players (source NCAA by Stacey J, US Today)*

however, that in this case the concept of the pyramid is geometrical not architectural, particularly in relation to Sydney Brenner's recent statement, 'we recognize the public myth that scientists are satisfied to be builders and that nobody's brick is better or bigger than anybody else's.'[25] Taking this argument much further is the refutation of the 'Ortega hypothesis' (Jose Ortega y Gasset) that 'experimental science has progressed thanks in large part to the work of men astoundingly mediocre, and even less than mediocre.' Based on a study of the citation practice of academic physicists, the sociologists Jonathan and Stephen Cole concluded that 'the data allow us to question the views stated by Ortega, Florey, and others that large numbers of average scientists contribute substantially to the advance of science through their research.[26] It seems, rather, that a relatively small number of physicists produce work that becomes the basis for future discoveries in physics. We have found that even papers of relatively minor significance have used to a disproportionate degree

159

the work of the eminent scientists.'[26] Similar results have also been reported in the discipline of sociology.[27]

If the above is true then it becomes important to determine whether there is any relation between the quantity and quality of information produced by scientists. de Solla Price in his book *Little Science, Big Science* observed: 'There is a reasonably good correlation between the eminence of a scientist and his productivity of papers. It takes persistence and perseverance to be a good scientist, and these are frequently reflected in a sustained production of scholarly writing.'[28] Furthermore, the proportion of prolific authors is relatively small; de Solla Price invokes the inverse square law, noting that 'for every 100 authors who produce one paper in a certain period there are 25 with two and 11 with three and so on.'[28]

In my own bibliographic work I became acutely aware of the quantity/quality question. Over 20 years ago we produced an exhaustive computerised bibliography of all the world's publications about a major global disease, from its discovery in 1852 to 1962.[29] Finding that the availability of that compendium did not satisfy our quest for useful information, copies of the bibliography were sent to about 50 of the world's experts to select all of the publications that they considered to be of importance and value. Of the 10 000 papers in the complete bibliography, 70% were not selected at all, 15% two or more times, and 345 six or more times. Using the latter as a basis, a core list of 404 papers was established by the experts. In the process of condensing each of these papers into a single volume[30] I learned that many of the 4% best articles in this list were scientifically and methodologically unsound.

This led to a major analysis of both the complete literature and that selected for quality, to ascertain whether means existed by which papers of quality could be identified.[22] The simple conclusion was that the best scientific and clinical papers tended to be produced by the best scientists, most of whom worked in the better institutions and published in the better journals. de Solla Price came to similar conclusions: 'Scientists tend to congregate in fields, in institutions, in countries, and in the use of certain journals. They do not spread out uniformly, however desirable that may or may not be. In particular, the growth is such as to keep relatively constant the balance between "the few giants" and "the mass of pygmies".'[28]

The body of clinical publications provides a recent example of how the vast quantity of information made available by computer is drastically reduced when considered in terms of both relevance and quality. The entire problem was shown in the Materials and

Methods section of the paper by Williamson *et al* reporting the results of their telephone survey on the use of information by clinicians (see above). To plan the design of their study they did an exhaustive and sophisticated MEDLINE search, which provided nearly 1000 citations. After they had carefully screened all of the titles only 150 papers were found to be relevant, in the sense of addressing the questions that the investigators were seeking to answer. On carefully reading each relevant paper the authors deemed only three of the 150 to be methodologically sound enough to be used in the design of their investigation.[19]

Of particular relevance to the glut of 'information' filling our libraries and databases are the autobiographical words of Charles Darwin: 'I happened to read for amusement Malthus' *On Population* and being well prepared to appreciate the struggle for existence which everywhere goes on from long continued observation of the habit of animals and plants, it at once struck me, that under these circumstances, favourable variations would tend to be preserved and unfavourable ones to be destroyed.' Years later, in 1859, Darwin published *On the Origin of the Species by means of Natural Selection, or the Preservation of Favoured Races in the Struggle for Life*. In terms of Darwinian evolution there is no system that I know of that has such a blatant disregard for the laws of natural selection and the preservation of favoured species as that of information.

Though Darwinian theory is contravened by the production and storage of information, it is vindicated by the use of the information by scientists and clinicians. Urquhart's study of 53 000 loan applications from the collection of 9120 periodicals in the British Lending Library for Science and Technology showed that more than half of the collection was never consulted and that a quarter was consulted only once. Half of the demand was satisfied by 40 journals, and 900 (10%) were sufficient to meet 80% of the requests.[31] A survey of interlibrary loans made by the National Library of Medicine found that of 37 000 serial titles, 88% were not borrowed once during the course of one year.[21] In a recent study at the great library of the Marine Biological Laboratories in Woods Hole, Massachusetts, which contains 5000 journal titles, 46% were not looked at once over the course of 10 months. Two per cent of the collection, 113 titles, accounted for fully half of the journal use, 10% for 80%, and 27% for 95%.[32] In the Allen Memorial Medical Library in Cleveland, which contains more than 3000 titles, only 300 were looked at in a period of one month, and only 120 frequently.[33] Despite the incontrovertible evidence that most of the

161

journal titles in libraries are not used and most of the remainder are consulted rarely, the Harris survey showed that biomedical scientists and clinicians believed that their libraries must be fully comprehensive.

As libraries are the paradigm for storing and obtaining information let us again turn to Margit Kraft. 'Academic libraries, particularly university libraries, are institutions whose purpose is to preserve, organize, and make accessible those graphic records that have contributed in the past and are contributing in the present to the advancement of knowledge. They are not institutions whose purpose is to preserve the output of the printing presses.'[21] From the scientific point of view the physicist Lewis Branscomb has observed: 'It is just as absurd for the user to tap the total collection of new material for his data as it would be for the jeweler to order 6 tons of gold-bearing ore when he wants to make a cufflink.'[34]

The coming alliance: human quality/machine quantity

For the past two decades or more we have been bombarded with the present and future capabilities of computers, electronic publishing, and artificial intelligence. It is about time that we add a unique capacity to the latter—that is, human intelligence. Jill Larkin approached this idea conceptually by addressing the human problems in handling large amounts of information, and discussed how 'computers might best help us to use our strengths and work around our weaknesses'.[6] A corollary would be how human intelligence might best help computers maximise their strengths and minimise their weaknesses.

Two acronyms define the computer: WYSIWYG (what you see is what you get) and GIGO (garbage in, garbage out). Regarding the latter, however, there is little doubt that if the computer were used as a refinery it should be possible to change GIGO to 'garbage in, gold out' (see the Branscomb cuff link analogy above).

In his book *Crisis in Communication* Sir Theodore Fox, renowned editor of the *Lancet*, noted in 1965 that, 'Machines cannot distinguish good papers from bad ones and have to treat all alike.'[35] Thus one unique aspect of human intelligence is the recognition of quality not only in music, art, and sports, but also in science. When Derek de Solla Price was discussing the quality of science in terms of the 'few giants' and the 'many pygmies' he noted that the latter keep 'wondering why it is that neither man nor nature pushes us toward egalitarian uniformity.'[25] This issue was discussed by the philosopher John Bruer as follows: 'the utopian concept allows us to elucidate a middle position between the best-science elitists and the populists. Both parties to that debate seize upon one aspect of the scientific enterprise and mistake that one aspect for the entirety of science. The populists are correct in arguing for egalitarianism and tolerance. These values are extremely important at the design stage of research. Science, however, does require a filtration process in which selectivity, criticism, and judgments of quality are extremely important. The best-science elitists are correct in upholding these values and the resulting meritocracy as part of the scientific enterprise. More important, having reached this middle position, it is but a short step to the justification of a selective approach to the scientific literature itself.'[36]

This takes us to de Solla Price's suggestion that the time may have come for a new approach, beyond abstracts, for the compression of information.[1] That new approach I submit is an emphasis on the small fraction of scientific and clinical information of quality and lasting value. Using an approach in which all published reports are entered into computerised databases, coupled with a hierarchical output system based on the quality of authors, journals, and papers using sophisticated citation analysis and other means of estimating quality, one can develop a far less time consuming and expensive means of obtaining scientific and clinical information of value. Beyond that one can search successive tiers of information, each of which increases exponentially in quantity while decreasing exponentially in quality.

In my own experience I had an opportunity to apply the bibliometrical principles I had been working on for years with the development of a programme at The Rockefeller Foundation called Coping with Biomedical and Health Information. We began with a meeting in 1979 in Bellagio, Italy, about medical libraries in the developing world, at which we learned that these institutions had for the most part declined to a virtually irretrievable level; in Latin America, for instance, 60% of all medical schools had essentially no libraries.[37] Using an intercommunication algorithm, William Goffman developed a comprehensive medical school library consisting of little more than 100 journals; 'use studies' such as those described above have shown that this small number of journals account for the most use in major medical libraries comprising 3000 journals. These journals were provided on microfiche, for ease and rapidity of shipping and for simplicity of storage and maintenance, plus reader-printers and the latest readers, to four medical schools in Indonesia, Egypt, Mexico,

163

and Colombia. All of the hardware and the journals and *Index Medicus* for six years cost a total of $50 000. In depth evaluation has shown a remarkable degree of use, and, in fact, regionalisation of most of the libraries.[83]

Several years later, because of our concern that ministries of health in the developing world did not have adequate access to data in determining their policies we developed a Comprehensive Information System in Health (CIShealth). The remarkable progress in technology enabled us to virtually provide complete and rapid access to global medical and health information systems. Using Goffman's algorithm, we provided a health library on microfiche consisting of five years of 69 journals in 29 subjects, accompanied by two advanced reader-printers. To this was added an IBM personal computer with a compact disc reader and MEDLINE on compact disc for five years, the latter providing access to all articles (including abstracts) in 3400 journals. The final item was a fax machine linked to an international document supply house with a limited amount of hard currency to buy articles after the approval of a trained 'gate keeper.' This system has been provided to the ministries of health of China, Zimbabwe, Mexico, and Brazil, at a total cost of $60 000 each.

My present position in a global communication and information organisation is related to the above endeavors. We are working at the integrative level involving journal and book publishing, on line databases and compact disc knowledge bases, and document delivery, all with an emphasis on the quality of our products. Concerning the access system to medical databases, our major concerns are with improving the efficiency of the search process with a transparent thesaurus to the 'medical subject headings,' a probablistic search system so that citations are printed in the order of their relevance, and (within that) a qualitative output in the order of the impact factors of the journals. Linked to this would be automatic document delivery within an hour from the most frequently ordered journals, either by modem or by fax.

Before proceeding to the concluding section of this chapter I would just like to summarise my views on electronic publishing. Robert Weber has presented what he calls potentially limiting factors in this area; I would call them opportunities. 'They involve the rate of new investment in advanced technologies, the rate at which the telephone system is upgraded, and the rate at which existing research networks are integrated into a national networking infrastructure. The next factor involves standards issues: standards for user interfaces and standards for text and images. The last two potential limitations involve advanced technology, specifically, whether photographic quality displays and printers will be developed and whether a workable means of enforcing copyright will be found.'[39] Frederick Bowes, until recently director of publishing of the *New England Journal of Medicine*, and one of the foremost thinkers and practitioners in the field of electronic publishing, has developed a concept of a 'digital warehouse' from which material can be produced in a wide variety of media, past, present, and future, and can be specifically tailored to a wide variety of special audiences. It is my belief that the elusive future of electronic publishing will soon be upon us.

A qualitative approach to medical publishing

In the past few years the use of qualitative input systems into biomedical and clinical books, reviews, newsletters, and journals has been gathering momentum.

Regarding books, the first wholly devoted to carefully evaluated clinical trials, *Effective Care in Pregnancy and Childbirth*, has recently been published by Oxford University Press.[40] A review in the *Lancet* which is entitled 'State of the obstetric art' describes the book in the following manner, 'Rather than the usual mixture of rewritten analyses and ex-cathedra statements that make up other large texts, it is based on formal analysis of evidence from controlled trials.'[41] A review in the *Medical Journal of Australia* began, 'It is a privilege to review what is arguably the most important publication in obstetrics since William Smellie wrote *A Treatise on the Theory and Practice of Midwifery* in 1752. This monumental collection and careful evaluation of all identifiable randomised clinical trials in obstetrics since 1950 is far more than a book. It is a triumph of impartial assessment over bias and a triumph of evidence based on numbers over opinions based on lack of experience.'[42]

In addition to the two volume work on perinatal medicine there is a condensed paperback version and a continuously updated database on floppy discs. The unique utility of the discs concerning the updating of meta-analyses, and the development of new such overviews is quite clear. However, it may also serve as a database for practising doctors, providing them with rapid, simple, unambiguous, and best-current-data for the care of their patients. At present we are working with Iain Chalmers and other top meta-analysts on expanding this system to all of clinical medicine under the rubric 'medical knowledge.'

In an article entitled 'Misinformation explosion: is the literature worth reviewing?' published in 1968, the physicist Lewis Branscomb emphasised the crucial role of scientific review articles, but only if the information reported was carefully sifted qualitatively. He described an analysis of 30 independent reports on helium ionisation cross section in which only 10% of papers had even rudimentary evidence concerning essential questions such as the prevention of secondary emission from the electron beam collector or the definition of the path length of the electrons in the ionising region.[34] A recent discussion of medical review articles by Mulrow echoed these concerns, beginning with, 'Good review articles are precious commodities.' This statement was made not only about their importance in helping individuals to obtain and absorb information efficiently, but also because they are rare, as most medical reviews are 'subjective, scientifically unsound, and inefficient.'[43] Mulrow then presented a systematic method for preparing a medical review article, which emphasised the formulation of a precise question, the use of efficient strategies for identifying relevant material of substantive quality and excluding irrelevant or poor quality material, and using standardised methods of appraising information.[43]

Scientists and physicians are coming to rely more and more on reviews and syntheses of published reports, such as those in the great Annual Review series which began over 60 years ago, many of which are at the top of the *Science Citation Index*. Nevertheless, if reviewers attempt a comprehensive survey of publications using even selected journals such as the 3400 in the MEDLINE files, their task becomes essentially impossible. One solution was found by Lionel Bernstein more than a decade ago in updating his viral hepatitis database. When the 10 experts involved did a search of MEDLINE over two and a half years they received 5700 citations, which they found impossible to handle. On going through many contemporary reviews they found that 80% of the articles cited were contained in only 18 journals; this reduced their task by about 90%.[44] Recently, a company called Current Science has developed a series of Current Opinion journals in clinical medicine and the biological sciences, which consist of concise authoritative reviews with selected annotated bibliographies that are updated annually. In the process of providing comprehensive bibliographies for the reviewers, they found that the high quality articles cited in the reviews came largely from relatively few journals (V Tracz, personal communication).

A new phenomenon is the development of newsletters summarising recent clinical information for doctors. *Journalwatch*, started by the Medical Publishing Group of the Massachusetts Medical Society, provides carefully crafted summaries of articles taken from about 20 selected clinical journals by a group of experts. Communication is completely electronic and the product is produced by desk top publishing techniques. An even more recent entry is the *ACP Journal Club* developed by Brian Haynes and associates at McMaster University, which is provided as a supplement to the *Annals of Internal Medicine*. Thirty eight journals are perused and articles are selected on the basis of pre-set criteria for presentation in the form of 'structured abstracts.' The selection criteria include random allocation or clearly identified comparison groups, at least 80% follow up, and use of an outcome measure of clinical importance. Review articles must have an identifiable Methods section and a statement of the criteria by which articles were selected for detailed review.[45]

And finally, on this occasion of the 150th anniversary of the *British Medical Journal*, I would like to discuss the clinical journal of the future in the context particularly of the four great weekly journals, which also include the *Journal of the American Medical Association*, the *Lancet* and the *New England Journal of Medicine*. Putting aside all of the issues of electronic publishing and communication, these remarks will be devoted to the basic issue of the content of these journals and how it is presented. When Thomas Wakley founded the *Lancet* in 1823 to 'incise the abscess on the medical body politic,' he planned to provide 'a correct description of all the important Cases that may occur, whether in England or on any part of the civilized Continent.'

One hundred and forty years later Wakley's distinguished successor, Sir Theodore Fox, presented his Heath Clark lectures on 'the functions and future of medical journals.'[35] He divided them into recorder journals and newspaper journals, with some serving both functions. The former 'records new observations and experiments and techniques. As one of the principal means of communication between investigators it is at present necessary for the advance of *medical knowledge*.' The function of the medical newspaper 'is to inform, interpret, criticise, and stimulate. . . . It is necessary for the advance of *medical practice*.' The four major weekly medical journals mentioned above all clearly fall into an intermediary group of recorder-newspapers.

Ole Harlem, for long editor of the *Norwegian Medical Journal*, in an article entitled 'Publish—but why perish?' refers to the 'ideal medical journal' as described by Arnold Relman, editor of the *New England Journal of Medicine*. This journal includes a core of technical information which all physicians share as well as the non-technical aspects of practice, reviews, and news of relevant social and political events. Harlem comments that 'ideals are important elements in our lives but we cannot live by them. . . . We have continued to cling to the publishing habits of our forefathers and have done nothing better than create one journal after another on more or less traditional lines.' He adds, 'The situation is indeed paradoxical. Instead of using modern information technology to create a contemporary medical information system we are using sophisticated techniques to shore up an obsolete system.'[46]

Recently, Brian Haynes has proposed a new kind of medical journal that would be specifically directed to practising doctors, whose information problems were so graphically described in the studies of Covell *et al*[18] and Williamson *et al*,[19] summarised above. Haynes ascribes part of the problem to the fact that most of the peer reviewed clinical journals communicate with several different audiences: from scientist to scientist (largely preliminary, uncontrolled studies), from scientist to practitioner (rigorous trials in clinical settings), from practitioner to practitioner (review articles), and from practitioner to scientist (case reports). Haynes recommends that journals should concentrate on specific audiences and proposes a new sort of clinical journal that would be devoted largely to rigorous trials and methodologically sound review articles that interpret the trials and their clinical applications.[47] This would decrease confusion among clinicians, and possibly even the media, between the fluid and rapidly changing reports of original biomedical communications and the more clinically relevant outcomes of large scale controlled trials, and particularly overviews of them.

I would agree with Haynes that journals of this kind are needed, but also believe that the ambiguity created by the structure of our major weekly 'recorder-newspaper' journals might be elucidated and obviated by the explicit division of their material into three, rather than the two general sections described by Fox. What are now called original articles should be clearly delineated into two separate sections. One called *scientific communications* would be devoted to scientists addressing their peers. Clinicians could and indeed should be encouraged to peruse this section in the clear understanding that they were participating in the intellectually stimulating frontiers of clinical and biomedical science. The other section might be labelled *clinical communications* and would cover the rigorous trials and overviews relevant to clinical practice that Haynes describes so eloquently. The important factor in the above dichotomy is to distinguish clearly to the practitioner and the public the important distinction between scientific and clinical communications. The third section would be the broad newspaper function described so well by both Fox and Relman.

Conclusion

This discussion began with the history of information technology from papyrus to parchment to paper to pixels, and then described the negative impact on medical education and practice of the ever more efficient production of information. Though recognising the enormous contribution of technology and the remarkable promise of the electronic age, which tantalisingly continues to hover on the horizon, I believe that the combination of human intelligence with the unique capabilities of computing machines will soon evolve into a true information and communication revolution. I share Robert Maxwell's belief that 'our scientific information system is at a watershed of technical, economic and social evolution'.[48] Technology for handling the quantity of information plus a human focus on its quality could be the next step in developing practical means of coping with this enormous problem. The plethora of medical information is preventing the remarkable developments of modern medicine from reaching their true recipients, the people for whom disease can either be prevented, cured, or ameliorated.

Coda

On this great occasion the last word should be given to Stephen Lock, an outstanding editor and a scholar in his profession. Almost a decade ago he wrote an editorial in the *BMJ* entitled 'Information overload: solution by quality?' The conclusion was, 'If, then, for biomedical journals the last twenty years has seen a preoccupation with questions of originality and ethics possibly the next twenty may be concerned with those of quality.'[49]

169

1 de Solla Price DJ. *Science since babylon*. New Haven, Connecticut: Yale University Press, 1961.
2 Rubin JS. Professional and scholarly publication in perspective. Presented to the Association of American Publishers meeting on professional and scholarly publishing, Washington DC, 2/90/90.
3 Lem S. *The cyberiad: fables for the cybernetic age*. New York: Avon, 1980.
4 Levi P. Full employment. *New Yorker*, April 23, 1990.
5 Greenes RA, Shortliffe EH. Medical informatics: an emerging academic discipline and institutional priority [special communication]. *JAMA* 1990;**263**:1114–20.
6 Larkin J. Information processing in scientific thought. In: Warren KS, ed. *Selectivity in information systems: survival of the fittest*. New York: Praeger, 1985;10–26.
7 Patel V, Evans DA, Groen GJ. Biomedical knowledge and clinical reasoning, In: Evans DA, Patel V, eds. *Cognitive science in medicine: biomedical modelling*. Cambridge, Massachusetts: MIT Press, 1989.
8 Schoolman H. Introduction to the future of information systems for the medical sciences. *Bull NY Acad Med* 1989;**65**:641–3.
9 Anonymous. Medical education: time for change. *J Am Board Fam Pract* 1990;**3**(suppl):1–65.
10 Tosteson DC. New pathways in general medical education. *N Engl J Med* 1990;**322**:234–8.
11 Bennet KJ, Sackett DL. Haynes RB, Neufeld VR, Tugwell P, Roberts R. A controlled trial of teaching critical appraisal of the clinical literature to medical students. *JAMA* 1987;**257**:2451–4.
12 Kennedy W, Warren K, Biscup R. Introducing students to the medical literature. *Med Educ* 1979;**13**:97–8.
13 Association of American Medical Colleges. *Medical education in the information age*. Washington DC: AAMC, 1986.
14 Yamamoto WS. 'Medical information science:' Insisting on a name can blunt its impact. *Med Inf (London)* 1984;**9**:195–7.
15 *World Congress on Medical Education*: Report, Edinburgh 1988. Edinburgh: World Federation of Medical Education, 1988.
16 Haynes RB, Davis DA, McKibbon A, Tugwell P. A critical appraisal of the efficacy of continuing medical education. *JAMA* 1984;**251**:61–3.
17 Evans CE, Haynes RB, Birkett NJ, Gilbert JR, Taylor DW, Sackett DL, *et al.* Does a mailed continuing education program improve physician performance? *JAMA*:1966;**255**:501–4.
18 Covell DG, Uman GC, Manning PR. Information needs in office practice: Are they being met? *Ann Intern Med* 1985;**103**:596–9.
19 Williamson JW, German PS, Weiss R, Skinner EA, Bowes F. Health science information management and continuing education of physicians. *Ann Intern Med* 1989;**110**:151–60.
20 Harris L and associates. *The future of information systems for the medical sciences*. New York: New York Academy of Medicine, 1987.
21 Kraft M. An argument for selectivity in the acquisition of materials for research libraries. *Library Quarterly* 1967;**37**:284–95.
22 Goffman W, Warren KS. *Scientific information systems and the principle of selectivity*. New York: Praeger, 1980.
23 Durack D. The weight of medical knowledge. *N Engl J Med* 1978;**298**:773–5.
24 Wyatt V. Swimming with the rising tide of research, *New Scientist* 1988(July);65–6.
25 Brenner S. The greatest satisfaction (book review). *Nature* 1990;**345**:675–6.
26 Cole JR, Cole S. The Ortega hypothesis. *Science* 1972;**178**:368–75.
27 Oromaner M. The Ortega hypothesis and influential articles in American sociology. *Scientometrics* 1985;**7**:3–10.
28 de Solla Price D. *Little science, big science*. New York: Columbia University Press, 1963.

29 Warren K, Newill V. *Schistosomiasis: a bibliography of the world's literature from 1852 to 1962.* Cleveland, Ohio: The Press of Western Reserve University, 1967.

30 Warren K. *Schistosomiasis: the evolution of a medical literature. Selected abstracts and citations 1852–1972.* Boston, Massachusetts: MIT Press, 1973.

31 Urquhart D. *Use of scientific periodicals.* (International Conference on Scientific Information.) Washington, DC: National Academy of Sciences-National Research Council, 1958;277–290.

32 Wolff A. A cold eye on mediocrity: filtering out the best of the biomedical literature. *RF Illustrated*, March 1986.

33 Goffman W. Morris T. Bradford's law and library acquisitions, *Nature* 1970;**266**:922–3.

34 Branscomb L. Misinformation explosion: is the literature worth reviewing? *Scientific Research* 1968;**3**:49–56.

35 Fox T. *Crisis in communication: the functions and future of medical journals.* London: Athlone, 1965.

36 Bruer J. Selectivity and the values of science, In: Goffman W, Bruer R, Warren K, eds. *Research on selective information systems.* New York: Rockefeller Foundation, 1980.

37 Saracevic T, ed. *Selective libraries for medical schools in less-developed countries.* New York: Rockefeller Foundation, 1980.

38 Saracevic T. Selective medical library on microfiche. *Bull Med Libr Assoc* 1988;**76**:44–53.

39 Weber R. The clouded future of electronic publishing. *Information Technology Quarterly* 1990;**9**:9–13.

40 Chalmers I, Enkin M, Keirse MJNC, eds. *Effective care in pregnancy and childbirth.* Oxford: Oxford University Press, 1989.

41 Lilford R. State of the obstetric art. [Book review of Chalmers I, Enkin M, Keirse M. *Effective care in pregnancy and childbirth.*] *Lancet* 1989;ii:1205–7.

42 MacLennan A. Obstetric milestone. [Book review of Chalmers I, Enkin M, Keirse M. *Effective care in pregnancy and childbirth.*] *Med J Aust* 1990;**152**:375–6.

43 Mulrow C. The medical review article: state of the science. *Ann Intern Med* 1987;**106**:485–8.

44 Bernstein L. The hepatitis knowledge base. In: Goffman W, Bruer R, Warren KS, eds. *Research on selective information systems.* New York: Rockefeller Foundation, 1980;72–105.

45 Haynes RB. The origins and aspirations of the ACP Journal Club [editorial]. *ACP Journal Club* supplement to *Ann Intern Med* Jan/Feb 1991; suppl 1: A18.

46 Harlem O. Publish—but why perish? In: *Swerving neither to the right nor the left.* London: Keynes Press, 1988;35–8.

47 Haynes RB. Loose connections between peer reviewed clinical journals and clinical practice. *Ann Intern Med* 1990;**113**: 724–8.

48 Maxwell R. *Dainton lecture.* Boston Spa: British Library, 1990.

49 Lock S. Information overload: solution by quality? *Br Med J* 1982;**284**:1289–90.

The position of paper in the emerging world of bioinformatics—could the journal be threatened?

JACK FRANKLIN

Research has traditionally ended in a primary article—a paper. As we all know this paper must follow a series of rules and guidelines for the presented research story to be understood, checked, and used in the continuing chain of work leading to greater scientific knowledge.

This end product is equally traditionally seen as *information*. Locating original papers of use to their research is an essential task in most scientists' lives and the majority therefore use bibliographic or secondary literature services such as MEDLINE (the online version of the MEDLARS information service from the National Library of Medicine) or EMBASE (the online version of the bibliographic database of Excerpta Medica, a division of Elsevier Science Publishers) to scan indexed abstracts to locate the primary article.

These databases are developed around the articles themselves (that is, they identify the subject matter that the article covers) but the information in these papers can also be used to build a number of other more specific databases as primary papers contain not only 'scientific stories' but summaries, digests, or edited versions of enormous amounts of other data and information, 'the results'. These results are increasingly being re-edited out of the primary text and placed in other (factual) databanks, often enriched or added to by the author (for instance the hybridoma databank for which the author is asked to add details on specificity, etc). Though a primary article is the final product of the research, increasingly the data on which the article's conclusions are drawn are also made available through other publicly accessible data services; we are approaching a situation whereby the individual parts of a research project are 'published' in a variety of products.

Databases are only as useful as their contents and the more complete they are the better. Until recently the builders of these specialist databases searched primary publications for relevant details and used these as their building blocks. However, it is clear that a large amount of data never reaches the finished journal article (some becomes irrelevant to the story in question but many editors just do not have the space for all the methodology and related ancillary information). There are therefore increasing cries for scientists to deposit their source cultures, cells, hybridomas, and codes, to name but a few, as well as descriptive information about them, in these databases and collections irrespective of whether they are relevant to a publication. Though some of these calls have come from scientists anxious to ensure that experiments can be repeated on the original material, the database producers have also emphasised how important it is for researchers to deposit cultures and data to ensure the above completeness. These calls have led to an enormous increase in the direct deposition of data and, for instance in the nucleotide sequence field, we now have up to 70% of the data arriving in this way. Thus there is an increasing separation between 'data' and the primary article.

These calls are not only from the righteous and self interested. Whereas research used to produce *information*, certain areas of research now actually depend on information technology and other peoples' data for their advance. It is this emerging area of bioinformatics, the merging of computer, information, and biomedical technology, that could challenge the publishing status quo.

Although bioinformatics has been advancing through biotechnology, medicine and medically related biological research is particularly affected because of the enormous effort being put into the various human and other genome projects.[1] Sequences have to be linked to genetic maps. The raw data in a gene sequence must be 'translated' into a (probably currently theoretical) protein. Such activities increasingly depend on the computer. Try aligning two nucleic acid sequences of a few thousand base pairs by hand to find the best 'fit'; if that does not convince you try identifying all the other sequences which might be like the one you deciphered yesterday—*without* a computer equipped with the specialist software. Scientists have estimated that the amount of data produced

173

during the human genome activities (three gigabytes of sequence data alone) will be so great that new techniques of data handling will have to be found before the data can be used (once the sequences are known and mapped; we have to work out how the proteins might look and then how they might work).

A few years ago the ubiquitous Vax was the only computer most biologists had heard of. Now larger mainframes, stretching up to supercomputers, are part of the biologists' armoury; and there are few topics for which the computer is not being used.[2] For instance, apart from its use in calculations, it is cheaper and swifter to prepare three dimensional models of drugs on a graphics machine than by spending months at the bench. And as microbial strains are increasingly classified on the basis of their media requirements, resistances, and sensitivities, so databases have to be searched to locate the individual strain that fits a user's requirements. Again, the reader of the primary paper must be spared this detail but the facts should be recorded for future use.

We are now seeing ways in which individual laboratory notebooks can be made available to other collaborators, making use of that enormous amount of data that does not itself warrant a primary article. Yet if it is stored in a usable, trustworthy, form it will become a real resource. At the same time, it could mean that the primary journal will no longer be the first step in the information dissemination chain. To avoid duplication and confusion these data will have to be integrated into the present information infrastructure, and so these databanks will become the equivalent of the present journals as far as the storage of factual information is concerned.

The database culture

The explosion in the number of biomedical journals is known to all, and there are very few research staff who can forgo a subscription to ISI's *Current Contents* or one of the newly launched electronic equivalents such as Excerpta Medica's *Medical Science Weekly*. Even so many relevant papers can still be missed, and so the use of abstract journals and their electronic brethren to 'check the literature' has increased in the past few years; in fact 'online searching', for most scientists and clinicians, means looking at EMBASE, BIOSIS, or MEDLINE for the references and abstracts that will lead them back to the paper they need for their further education and research.

We also have a growing number of biomedical factual databanks;

there are even databases describing databases (LiMB (listing of information sources in molecular biology) and DBIR database on biotechnology information resources) and these are increasingly available on computers linked via the commercial and academic telecommunication networks. Though the searching of secondary sources was the domain of information professionals, factual, structural, and other 'scientific' databases need to be searched by the researchers themselves. This requires at least a modicum of information technology skill, but most of the scientists involved are au fait with the electronic mail technology required. At the same time the international academic networks are presently being upgraded to carry vast amounts of data extremely swiftly, and gateways between them mean that it is becoming easier to cross from one network to another in the same way that a letter is passed from one postman to another—only that this occurs without a perceptible pause. We can now easily search a computer situated across the world, or 'chat' with a similarly placed colleague through a computer terminal, a modem, and the telephone services.

It is therefore no surprise to find specific services being established to enable like-minded scientists to communicate with each other and to access data sources. Thus in the UK, SEQNET (a nucleic acid based series of databases carried on the SERC Daresbury computer and made available, with supporting software, to academic and industrial customers) was established to provide molecular biologists with the various databases they require (nucleotide sequences, protein sequences, genetic maps, etc). Currently run by the SERC, the service offers a central computer where the various relevant molecular biology databases are mounted. SEQNET is also linked to the EMBL (European Molecular Biology Laboratory) Data Library as it is a node of EMBnet, a communications network whereby users can access the EMBL computer for updates of their various nucleotide sequence files. Thus the UK users receive nightly updates of those data as well as being able to deposit their own results in the library by this means; although floppy discs and other Email services are also available. Users of SEQNET have formed a closed user group that keeps them in touch with their national peers while also providing them with international databases in a prepackaged format.

Another service, established for microbiologists, is the Microbial Strain Data Network (MSDN) which connects users to various culture collections and related databases and runs on the commercial Telecom Gold electronic mail service.[3] This not only allows members to write to each other but also links them to a variety of different culture collections such as: in the USA the American Type Culture Collection, in Germany the Deutschen Sammlung von Mikroorganismen, the British Porton establishment, and many other collections based inside individual institutes or departments. The MSDN takes the user to the relevant computer to search that data for information or products. If the user locates what he requires, he can order it immediately and receive the bill when he receives his monthly invoice from the MSDN. Again, the closed user group benefits from its mutual interests, but this service offers future providers of information a profiled audience with an efficient means of access.

Direct deposition

These developing databases are at present (often) rudimentary and based on data gleaned from the primary publications. All too often they have been developed by scientists to serve a specific role and less attention has been paid to structure and dissemination. At the same time many others are now very sophisticated and both GenBank (an American nucleic acid sequence databank produced in conjunction with the EMBL service) and EMBL have developed advanced techniques for data collection, collation, and storage. They are currently encouraging the direct deposition of nucleic acid sequences by asking authors to deposit data direct into the databanks. This increases the speed of collection and the content, and therefore the use of the bank, but it also means that the material being deposited in these databank(s) is being 'uncoupled' from the primary publication; it will also not have been submitted to the traditional methods of evaluation—that is, peer review.

This lack of refereeing is seen by many as a serious deterrent to depositing data. But direct deposition is not a 'soft option' for the author: it is impossible just to 'send in a floppy' and hope that it can be read by the receiving centre. The EMBL Data Library has produced error checking and validation software which helps their authors follow the necessary rules to avoid disasters. This offers the start of peer reviewing: just as editors can refuse a paper on the grounds of style and make up, so database managers can ensure that the data has been prepared within standard guidelines. Once in the database the information is available for review and users can use the electronic mail networks to voice their concerns and questions. If storage costs continue to fall this might be the ultimate reviewing service—let everyone look at the data and comment accordingly.

We therefore have a situation in which data are being collected for a variety of factual databases and is becoming available for third party examination and use outside the traditional journal. These moves also provide an opportunity for interaction and comment in an interactive forum—already one centre in Paris allows authors to deposit nucleic acid sequence data for 'informal use and examination' prior to the same data being written up or deposited in the EMBL.

These communities are already computer dependent. The computer is essential in the recording of information and in its manipulation. The user community is connected together via a network. Why bother with paper at all?

Will electronic information catch on?

I hope that everyone agrees that the journal's main activity is to provide information in an educated and accurate manner.

I left academic life for the commercial world 17 years ago. On my arrival in a major publishing house I spent a few days 'learning the ropes' from a very well respected (computer) publisher who informed me that journals would be dead within five years; taken over by computers and networks. My company now publishes *Scientific Serials Review*—a journal reviewing new titles in biomedicine—and we regularly cover 75–100 new titles each year; thus the time scale of my doom-ridden friend's prediction was somewhat out. (The growth in titles and papers is difficult to estimate but most estimates agree that it is around 10% a year—at a time when library budgets, although no longer being cut, are still not growing.)

This explosion in the number of titles means that few libraries can hold all the relevant titles their constituents require. Whereas a few years ago most librarians spoke of holding 70% of their requirements, many are now satisfied if they hold 60%, or even less.

If we look at these journals, most arise because scientists want to concentrate and exchange their efforts and knowledge among a small peer group of similarly interested experts. The role of the publisher is to package and disseminate this information. However, though I have heard many society and commercial publishers extolling their own virtues, they are ignoring—or forgetting—the fact that the scientific journal is part of the peculiar *the-author-is-the-editor-is-the-referee-is-the-purchaser-is-the-reader* circle.

Despite this interdependence, the market for primary publications is dominated by 'expensive journals'. A great many, if not the vast majority, of authors would probably be willing to see their data made available cheaply to their own peer group, as many openly resent the role that (commercial) publishers now play. Some societies have indeed established journals to break out of the commercial circle (although others have announced their intention to publish titles for profit and the good of their members) but, almost inevitably, if the subject is worth a good journal then the journal is pronounced as being required reading outside the original group that established it. So in comes the publisher to ensure that the title is properly marketed, distributed, and managed, and up go the costs.

But the *original* need was to communicate with a peer group. The first journals required a change in mentality and distribution techniques when they appeared in place of the learned book, and we could now be at a similar crossroads. Electronic networks offer the present generation a seemingly cheap (most academic networks are subsidised and the individual user pays very little, if anything, for communication) method of communication. Furthermore, these networks are already used for accessing factual and secondary information—only the exchange of primary information remains to be done.

As indicated above, once a scientist is attached to a network, has mastered the technology, and is in contact with like minded scientists, the inclination to use the network instead of the post is great. Many of the problems of post disappear. Electronic mail arrives instantaneously. Answers can be requested politely. Messages (from notes to full papers) can be distributed to one, two, a selection, or all users of a service. Data can be sent in a machine-readable form to be used by other colleagues. Users can collate data, compare services, etc, etc. So why not use databases as replacements for journals?

The bridge between networks and journals

Specific data networks with publishing features are being developed. The newly developed MSDN already offers 450 microbiologists throughout the world the chance to communicate with each other and search a variety of databases and databanks. They now seek out and order a variety of specific cultures, and soon they will also have access to pieces of news and bulletin boards; so why not a journal?

Commercial experiments have certainly been tried. The first biomedical journal to appear in both paper and electronic formats was Elsevier's *IRCS Medical Science*.[4][5] This was followed by numbers of experiments in the early '80s when the full text of the research article was mounted on two database hosts.[6-8] The database was built by converting published texts by optical character recognition or retyping (still probably the most cost efficient). Electronic channels were established to accept papers 'online' but few were received, mainly because it was far too early for the word processor to have made its impact on departmental offices, which meant that there were no 'electronic manuscripts' in the first place. The service worked as far as the technology was concerned but it was obvious that there were far too few 'medical users' online to use the full text service (unlike an abstract service, full text is best used by the reader or user).

Another interesting project was *Clinical Notes Online* produced in the middle 1980s. Doctors were asked to submit clinically responsible case studies to be mounted in a database. These were mounted on Datastar and on a private bulletin board. We gained a group of converts but unfortunately insufficient to make it pay (although interestingly I now believe that it would have survived on an academic network). We had to produce a paper edition to satisfy university authorities that a 'publication' had occurred, and an interesting development was that occasionally *we* produced a paper that the authors had submitted to the Email file.

There have been many similar experiments in the USA. The American Medical Association has its own Email and data services system—AMANET. COLLEAGUE, the medical information service owned by the online company, BRS, runs bulletin boards and has recently taken over the MEDLINK medical library service established by the Medical Publishers Group (previously owned by the publishers of the *New England Journal of Medicine*). We are now also seeing increasing numbers of 'private' databases in which, for example, major clinical trials are being run with the help of networks.

Recognition

The major drawback to putting good science into anything other than a recognised journal is reduced recognition. Authors still have to publish or perish. Many universities, institutes, and granting bodies still measure the quality of research on its final resting place in the learned journals and not on its real value to the scientific community. The many excuses for this are well known but it remains true that we live in an era when any self respecting author tries to gain recognition by publishing a highly cited journal.

In itself, this should cause no problem. The electronic medium should lend itself to more sophisticated methods of scientific evaluation than 'each paper is seen by 2·5 referees' (that is, the first two referees disagreed). For instance, though it is impossible to gauge exactly what articles are read in a journal, it is very easy to register how many times a full paper is downloaded (read) from a database. A 'rating form' could also be added to the end of an (electronic) article. When monitoring the use of *Clinical Notes Online* we were able to see which papers attracted the most interest. We confirmed that adventurous titles pay off in terms of initial interest, but we could also see for how long people accessed each file and in that way estimate the degree of real interest in that article. And we managed to persuade one 'granting body' that a 'publication' in this service warranted the author at least a few 'brownie points.'

Another parallel trend that might help this acceptance is the increasing use of document delivery to satisfy the user. The biomedical discipline generates a particularly strong demand for document delivery and the ADONIS project, for which some 350 biomedical journals are stored on CD-ROMs so that individual articles can be sent to order, is a major move in this direction. This service is presently using analogue storage of the pages, but it is just as simple to store the text digitally as a byproduct of the final, accepted, electronic paper. This could open the door for the electronic journal, produced firstly as a byproduct of the paper journal but later as a direct transfer of the digital file.

Finance

Another problem restricting electronic publishing advances at the present time is that these systems do not generate a means for earning money (Franklin J. The commercialisation of bioinformatics. First Canadian bioinformatics meeting, Ottawa, 1989.) The main users of such factual databanks are academics. Though the computer and communication infrastructure for such services is expensive, subsidies in the form of central payments for such infrastructures mean that the user pays very little; in many cases nothing. Yet any 'commercial' service, and these will be needed if the systems are to be accepted and run with a professional infrastructure, would not have these subsidies and so could not recover the required investment at the same price levels. This will cause resistance—people always assume that information is cheap—and so reduce the advance of such database developments.

Nevertheless, the MSDN service is starting on a commercial basis. Unit costs have been kept low because of the efficiency of the service, and users may be the first to be ready to switch to using the computer for other types of information.

Another financial problem could really be quite advantageous to users. Electronic databases allow them to search first for the material required. In practice users buy only what they need, unlike readers of journals which include many papers that the subscriber might never read. The profitability of journals is often related to this fact, which is a major reason that many commercial companies are less enthusiastic about electronic databases. (In a study carried out for the European Commission in 1987/88 we found only one commercial publisher actually researching such services; another, very senior, executive openly 'hoped that the electronic revolution won't come'.[10] Ultimately we will have to think up new financial models for our scientific information, and the electronic age will probably have to wait for that moment before coming 'of age'.

Conclusions, or do I believe it will happen?

The above indicates that we could, today, establish electronic journals. These might be based on the traditional journal model, but they might also have several refinements that would add to the efficiency and the use of that information. These movements/trends appear to me to offer the information world new opportunities.[11] Select groups (markets) require specific information. They do not want to have to wade through vast amounts of different publications in media and, using as they do electronic media for much data gathering, they could move to electronic services for their 'published information'.

Of course, people are then technology dependent, though paper is still a superb medium for the written word and a 'lap-top' is no use for accessing an online file on a train (although there are those who say it can be done).

Because electronic publishing is possible, people committed to electronic systems, and there are many, tend to assume that paper journals will disappear. But this technology provides an additional, not substitute, medium. It enhances communication, it allows data to be transferred in manipulable formats, and people can use the services to examine several (distributed) sources at one sitting. But there will still be a need for journals, and scientists are already writing papers after reviewing electronic data. (I have recently read a preprint, sent by Email, of an article that analyses the links between hybridomas and nucleic acid sequences. The data were gleaned from databanks but the intellectual effort was easy to judge, and the paper will make good reading for a variety of scientists).

At the moment, and because electronic services are technology driven, the user communities are still too small for a general widespread bombardment of electronic information. Such services will begin in disciplines such as bioinformatics where the computer network is part of the science, and gradually we will see groups emerging who use electronic mail services to discuss 'papers'. At the same time, because these services are computer driven, there will be some people who refuse to use them. But that presents no problem. Those people can use the paper printouts of electronic files. We can also accept their floppy discs rather than their manuscripts for production.

Postscript

These same people will probably counter by claiming that they need the illustrations. Therefore, finally, I would like to make a comment on 'pictures'. I have now spent more than 10 years researching these types of problems. Ten years ago I was part of a team looking at the use of full text as an alternative to the paper journal. We created a database of some 24 000 pages and mounted this for full text retrieval. We studied its use in 33 universities in the USA and Europe and, from the start, we learnt that *everyone* was sure the experiment was doomed because of the lack of illustrations. When we revisited the sites no-one referred to this point. Nowadays, with the increasing use of faxes and photocopying, illustration quality is so poor that only those scientists who require glossy prints need worry; and they can receive them by courier if needed. In the future, those people will receive their required illustrations beamed down through satellite links to high definition televisions at off-peak viewing time. But that is another technology and time.

1 Benson D, Boguski M, Lipman DJ, Ostell J. The National Centre for Biotechnology Information. *Genomics* 1990;6:
2 Berendsen HJC. *A bioinformatics workstation*. Brussels, Belgium: Commission of the European Communities, 1986.
3 Kirsop B. Microbial Strain Data Network: a service to biotechnology. *International Industrial Biotechnology*, 1988;8:24–7.

4 Buckingham M, Franklin J, Westwater J. IRCS moves into electronic publishing. *IRCS Medical Science* 1982;**10**:276.

5 Buckingham MCS, Franklin J, Westwater J. *IRCS online: experiences with the first electronic biomedical journal.* Proceedings Seventh International Online Information Meeting. Oxford: Learned Information, 1983:105–10.

6 Franklin J. Primary information online in biomedicine—a short appraisal. *Scholarly Publishing* 1982;**13**:

7 Franklin J. *Biomedical journals online.* Proceedings Sixth International Online Information Meeting. Oxford: Learned Information, 1982:210–7.

8 Franklin J, Buckingham MCS, Westwater J. *Biomedical journals in an online full text database: a review of reaction to ESPL.* Proceedings Seventh International Online Information Meeting. Oxford: Learned Information, 1983:407–10.

9 Franklin J. *The future of bioinformatics—commercial developments. Biotechnology Information '86.* (Proceedings of meeting, 1985, Sussex.) Oxford: IRL Press, 1987.

10 Franklin J. *The role of information technology and services in the future competitiveness of Europe's biology based industries.* Brussels: Commission of the European Communities, 1988.

11 Anonymous. *Bioinformatics in Europe 1—Strategy for a European biotechnology information infrastructure.* Brussels: European Federation of Chemical Industries (CEFIC), 1990.

PART 5
THE FUTURE

Through the crystal ball darkly: medical journals and the future

RICHARD SMITH

'Radio has no future,' 'heavier than air flying machines are imposs-ible,' and 'x rays will prove to be a hoax.' These are three of the predictions made by Lord Kelvin when he was president of the Royal Society from 1890 to 1895.[1] Lord Kelvin is by no means alone in being wildly wrong with his predictions (see box),[1] and those who sit down to write about the future should keep these errors at the front of their minds.

Wrong predictions

'Everything that can be invented has been invented.'—The director of the US Patent Office, 1899

'Television won't last. It's a flash in the pan.'—Mary Somerville, pioneer of radio educational broadcasts, 1948

'Democracy will be dead by 1950.'—John Langdon-Davis, *A Short History of The Future*, 1936.

'There is no likelihood that man can ever tap the power of the atom.'—Robert Mullikan, Nobel Prize winner, 1923

'As a work of art, it is naught.'—The *New York Times* review of Bizet's *Carmen*, 1878

'A hundred years from now it is very likely that *The Jumping Frog* alone will be remembered.'—Harry Thurston Peck on the works of Mark Twain, 1901

Predicting the future has often been the job of frauds and shamans, but Americans are interested enough in the future to put *Megatrends 2000: Ten New Directions for the 1990s*[2] at the top of the *New York Times* bestseller list for many weeks.

We don't want to know too much about the future—for instance, to be able to read our genes and know when we will die and of what disease—but we are fascinated to take a peek. Hence the Palo Alto public library has about a dozen books on the future including one that makes predictions like: '2086, the first biochip, a superconductor made of protein, is implanted into the brain of a 63 year old California security guard'; and '2100 the first completely robotic penis is fashioned out of real human flesh and electronic components.'[3]

So if the future is unpredictable and the province of cranks should we forget it and get on with the present? I think not. Surveys of organisations[4-6] and countries[7] suggest that it is those who look to the future who excel. Those driven by tactics rather than strategy fail, and medicine has not distinguished itself as a profession by its planning. Doctors are propelled by science and suffering and rarely seem to know where they are aimed. Hence a glance to the future may be useful. Here I want to say a little about the pleasures and dangers of futurology and then look at the future in general, the future of medicine, and the future of medical publishing—relating these all the time to the future of medical journals.

Studying the future

The discipline of futurology enjoyed popularity in the 60s and 70s but has now declined. But it has not disappeared; rather people from many disciplines look to the future without calling themselves futurists or futurologists. There has always been a wild, slightly crazy side to futurology, but there are also sober groups of researchers using thorough techniques rather than crystal balls and hunches. One essential element of respectable futurology well described by Roy Amara, the immediate past president of the Institute for the Future, is to recognise the pre-eminence of long term trends over passing fads. Most of us are inclined to overestimate the impact on the future of short term trends and underestimate the importance of long term trends.[8]

Those who look to the future have a tendency to gravitate towards either optimism or pessimism—and maybe this tendency arises almost mathematically when you project your observations of the moment. Thus the popular *Megatrends* has an air of heady optimism, whereas many of the writers on the environmental future tend to the apocalyptic.[9] [10] These writers follow long traditions with Plato, Thomas More, Karl Marx, Joachim of Floris, and Edward Bellamy[11] on the side of the Utopians; Malthus, Fairfield Osborn,[12] George Orwell,[13] and the Club of Rome[14] on the side of the catastrophists; and Aldous Huxley on both sides.[15] [16]

Futurologists use many techniques but usually begin with *trend extrapolation*, which projects into the future what has been happening recently. In some circumstances this will be useful, but it has led to many errors.[17] Still more dangerous may be *forecasting by analogy*. Much more popular is what has been called *genius forecasting* in which a bright well informed person examines the present and then makes judgements about the future. Herman Kahn[18] and Daniel Bell,[19] who coined the term postindustrial and is the intellectual father of *Megatrends*, are examples of genius forecasters.

Another method is to use the *Delphi technique*, whereby experts are asked for opinions on the future which are then tabulated and fed back anonymously to the same experts. Amara, one of the people who developed the technique, has observed, however, that the technique is slow, expensive, and blunt.[9] Much more popular these days is the more informal *scenario setting*, which is a 'description of an internally consistent, plausible future.'[8] One reason that scenario setting is popular is that it does not purport to be a prediction but simply puts forward some intelligent ideas that can be used as a basis for discussion with those who need to think about the future.

Ferkiss has reviewed the outcome of the forecasts of futurologists and found some spectacular mistakes:[17] 'We are now founding colleges at the rate of 20 or more a year,' said a Ford Foundation expert in the mid-60s, 'and I believe in ten years we will be founding them at the rate of one a week.'[20] (I write this at Stanford in a week that this prestigious university has had to dip twice into its waiting list to reach enough undergraduates.) Futurologists have tended to begin with science, technology, and economics, working on the idea that these are the developments that drive social and political change. Generally, says Ferkiss, predictions of scientific breakthroughs—particularly in the biological sciences—have been overstated, perhaps because scientists tend towards optimism. Economic predictions are little better, and educational, social, and political predictions are often even more wrong. Very few people, for instance, saw that the Berlin Wall was about to come down.

TABLE I — *The characteristics of a postindustrial society as predicted by Bell*[20]

1 The centrality of theoretical knowledge
2 The creation of a new intellectual technology – for instance, computer driven linear programming and Markov chains
3 The spread of a knowledge class
4 The change from goods to sevice
5 A change in the character of work – to primarily 'a game between persons'
6 The role of women – for example, increasing participation in the labour force
7 Science as the imago – the absorption of science into new institutions
8 Situses as political units – vertical orders may become more important than horizontal units
9 Meritocracy
10 The end of scarcity?
11 The economics of information – information is by its nature a collective not a private good

But at the end of his short and fascinating monograph Ferkiss argues that people have little choice but to look to the future: 'their only choice is between being completely surprised by the future and therefore wholly subject to the control of external forces or, alternatively, having some basis of knowledge about what is possible so that they can attempt to shape the future in accord with their own desires and values. The choice is . . . between complete unfreedom and relative freedom.'[17]

The general future

Table I shows what Bell called 'the new dimensions of a postindustrial society',[19] whereas table II shows the 'megatrends' of the 80s and table III the 'megatrends' of the 90s.[2] Naisbitt and Aburdene define megatrends as 'large social, economic, political, and technological changes [that] are slow to form, and once in place . . . influence us for some time—between seven and ten years or longer.' These trends may, the authors admit, 'seem a little too arbitrary,' but they do provide a starting place and they do, I believe, seem to capture something important. Thus Bell says that 'the two large dimensions of a postindustrial society . . . are the centrality of theoretical knowledge and the expansion of the service sector as against a manufacturing economy.' These are trends that are well established in Britain, the United States, and other developed economies—and they augur well for medical journals, which trade in theoretical knowledge for one of the largest parts of the service economy.

Something that neither of these books mentions much, however,

TABLE II — *The megatrends of the 80s (Naisbett and Aburdene[2])*

1 Industrial society to information society
2 Forced technology to high technology
3 National economy to world economy
4 Short term to long term
5 Centralisation to decentralisation
6 Institutional help to self help
7 Representative democracy to participatory democracy
8 Hierarchies to networking
9 North to south
10 Either/or to multiple option

is the environment. But that it seems to me is where any discussion of the future must start. Many of the catastrophists believe that disaster may arrive quickly if we don't all begin to do something to improve the environment.[9]

POPULATION GROWTH

The pressures on the environment begin, argue the Ehrlichs, with population: 'Global warming, acid rain, depletion of the ozone layer, vulnerability to epidemics, and exhaustion of soils and groundwater are all . . . related to population size.'[9] The rate of population growth has slowed since 1970, but because the decline has been gradual the increments continue to grow larger. Table IV shows how the annual increase in world population was 84 million during the 80s but will be 96 million (a country about the size of Mexico each year) during the 90s. The population will be about 6·25 billion in the year 2000, and the developing world will not reach a steady state until the middle of the next century. Table V shows the countries that will gain over 20 million people between 1988 and 2000.[21] This list consists almost entirely of poor countries, and population growth will keep those countries poor.

TABLE III — *The megatrends of the 90s (Naisbett and Aburdene[2])*

1 The booming global economy of the 1990s
2 A renaissance in the arts
3 The emergence of free market socialism
4 Global lifestyles and cultural nationalism
5 The privatisation of the welfare state
6 The rise of the Pacific rim
7 The decade of women in leadership
8 The age of biology
9 The religious revival of the new millennium
10 The truimph of the individual

TABLE IV — *Growth in world population by year and decade (source: Worldwatch[10])*

Year	Population (billions)	Increase by decade (millions)	Average annual increase
1950	2·515		
1960	3·019	504	50
1970	3·698	679	68
1980	4·450	752	75
1990	5·292	842	84
2000	6·251	959	96

Medical journals have a duty to remind their readers of these facts, which they roughly know but constantly put to the back of their minds. Much work remains to be done on birth control methods, and medical journals will publish some of that work.

POVERTY

In 1989 the world had 157 dollar billionaires, about two million millionaires, and about 100 million homeless.[10] About 400 million people are undernourished and two billion drink and bathe in water contaminated with pathogens. Some 12 million children die every year of malnutrition or diarrhoea, and the World Bank and the United Nations Food and Agriculture Organisation estimate that between 700 million and one billion people live in absolute poverty. The figure shows how the rich are getting richer while the income

TABLE V — *Countries that will gain over 20 million in population between 1988 and 2000 (population in millions) (source: Institute for the Future[21])*

Country	1988	2000	Increase
India	817	1013	196
China	1088	1242	154
Nigeria	112	161	49
Brazil	151	195	44
Indonesia	184	227	43
Pakistan	107	145	38
Bangladesh	110	144	34
Soviet Union	286	311	25
Ethiopia	48	71	23
Philippines	63	86	23
United States	246	268	22
Iran	52	74	22
Vietnam	65	86	21
Mexico	84	104	20

of the poorest has hardly risen at all—meaning that the gap has grown substantially.[10] Almost certainly poverty increased dramatically in 1989, and over 40 developing countries ended the 80s poorer in per caput terms than when they began.[10]

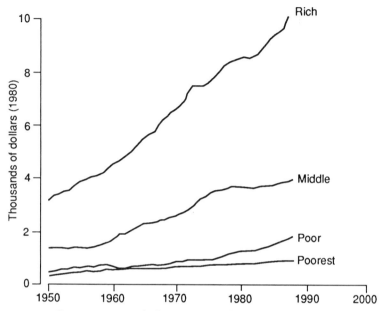

FIGURE —*Income per person in four categories of countries (source: Worldwatch[10])*

Lack of productive assets, physical weakness and illness, rapidly expanding population, massive debt (in 1989 the developing world owed about $1.2 trillion—half its collective gross national product), trade protectionism in developed countries, capital flight, and falling prices for their exports combine to make it likely that many of the world's poor will stay that way in the '90s.

Medical journals will continue to publish on the diseases of poverty and contribute to the search for ways to lessen the disease load of the poor—both through technological development and better health policy. The World Health Organisation estimates that increasing annual investment in preventive care by 75 cents for each person in the developing world would save five million lives a year. Journals also need to investigate ways to make their information available in an affordable form to health workers in the developing world.

193

HUNGER

World food production grew dramatically between the '50s and the '80s but in the past half decade has stalled.[10] Why? The answer seems to be a growing scarcity of new cropland and fresh water, the lack of any new technologies, and the effects of planetary degradation on food production. At least two of these three factors seem set to continue.

Medical journals cannot feed the world, but they can contribute to the analysis of the causes of hunger and the routes to reversing it. In addition, worldwide movements of doctors—like International Physicians for the Prevention of Nuclear War—have increasingly turned their attention to global issues like hunger. Medical journals will cover their campaigns.

ENVIRONMENTAL PROBLEMS

Concern about environmental problems is rightly growing rapidly. In the United States membership of environmental organisations has increased from under one million in 1970 to over five million in 1989, and the number of Green seats in the European Parliament increased from none in 1979 to 39 (7·5% of the total) in 1989.[21]

Global warming is perhaps the potentially most catastrophic of the environmental changes. Whether the warming of 0·3°C–0·6°C seen so far this century is the result of greenhouse gases is disputed, but there is agreement from the many computer models constructed of future temperatures that warming will continue. The Intergovernmental Panel on Climatic Change predicted in May 1990 from its 20 or so models that world temperature will rise by between 2·4°C and 5·1°C by 2070.[22] Its best bet was a rise of 3·0°C, which would mean a rise in sea level of 45 cm. The computer models are crude and have substantial problems with, for instance, predicting the effects of cloud cover, and working out how warming will vary regionally and seasonally. They do, however, agree that there will be warming, but whether there will be widespread flooding of world cities and massive famine because of desertification is unclear.

What must be recognised is that a quarter of the world's population accounts for 70% of the world's carbon emissions based on fossil fuels.[9] Thus China currently has a per caput consumption that is 7% of that of the United States. The hugeness of the Chinese population means that a doubling of its per caput use of coal by the year 2000 (and it presently plans greater increases) would more than offset the US ceasing to use coal altogether.[9] Roughly the same

194

increase would be achieved by India increasing its per caput consumption to what China's is today.

Depletion of the ozone layer is a problem that has led to rapid international action that may serve as a model for future international cooperation. That chlorofluorocarbons might cause a decline in global ozone was predicted in 1974, and in 1982 unusual depletions were seen over Antarctic. The 'ozone hole' was clear by 1985, and the first international agreement on reducing production of chlorofluorocarbons was reached at Montreal in 1987. By May 1989 agreement had been reached among 80 nations to end production and use of the chemicals by the year 2000. Nevertheless, the UK stratospheric ozone review group expects ozone depletion to continue for a while, and there are likely to be increases in skin cancer and cataracts and serious disturbances to the world's ecosystem.[23]

Global warming and depletion of the ozone layer are the two environmental problems attracting the most attention at the moment, but there are also serious problems with air and water pollution, deforestation, acid rain, and disposal of solid waste.[10] Doctors have played a crucial part in the story of air pollution but have been much less prominent in the debates on other environmental issues. The *BMJ* has in the past couple of years published articles on greening the NHS[24] and the possible effects on health from the thinning of the ozone layer,[25] but doctors and general medical journals must have a much larger contribution to make to the environmental debate. A study of articles on the environment in three influential US newspapers showed a virtual doubling in numbers between 1981 and 1989, and a much bigger increase must be likely in the next decade.[21]

A GLOBAL ECONOMY

World trade is growing rapidly, and in an increasing number of industries you either become a global competitor or die.[26 27] The pace of growth has been increased by a host of factors: the continuing fall in trade barriers; the convergence of management and technological skills accompanied by rapid diffusion of technology; improvements in international communication (Americans made 580 million minutes of overseas calls in 1977 and 4·7 billion minutes in 1987,[2] and American businesses are predicted to double their use of long distance calls by 2000[28]); the opening up of Eastern Europe; the emergence of fast growing economies in Asia; and the growth of strong international competitors.

The leading medical journals have been international for a long time, and 20 years ago medical academics probably travelled more than most business people. But the future may be that medical journals will need to become still more international to be successful, and the future may see little space for journals that do not look much beyond their own shores. Life is also likely to become increasingly difficult for those journals not published in English.

THE WORKPLACE

Organisations are changing. Those that are successful are becoming less hierarchical, more specialist, more dependent on information, more flexible, and faster changing.[29] The organisations of the future will be constantly rebuilt and rearranged, and employees will find themselves working predominantly in teams with a different group of people for each project. Employees will work more flexibly in that they will often work from home for more of their time, often job share or work part time, and increasingly keep haphazard hours.[30] Electronic linkages will be more important and commuting less important. And these new organisations will be built around learning. 'Organisations that can be self critical—and can learn to keep improving on today's work while aggressively preparing for tomorrow's—will be more successful than those organisations that evolve towards greater stability and complacency.'[31]

Medical journals have tended to be flat organisations anyway and they may find it easier than many organisations to adapt to the future. But most medical journals have not had a strong tradition of people working in teams, and they have had a tendency to keep people in boxes—particularly in editorial versus business boxes. The future may well see young doctor editors learning and working in marketing or international promotion. And, although editorial work might lend itself to flexible work patterns and electronic linkages, this is not yet widely seen—but surely will be.

THE RISE OF WOMEN

The need for new organisations is driven by the nature of the tasks to be accomplished, by technology, and by the needs of employees. One group who particularly need flexibility in their work are women who want to have children. In 20 years' time many men will probably also benefit from being able more easily to combine career and family, but for the next 10 years it will be woman who benefit most. And organisations that are flexible enough to be able to recruit and keep women will be at a competitive advantage—for the competition for skilled workers, an increasing proportion of whom will be women, will increase.[32] Provision of day care facilities is likely to become a key competitive factor in the next decade, and the *Wall Street Journal* is predicting that some companies will soon be offering breast feeding breaks.[28]

Half of British medical graduates are now women, and the last four doctors appointed to the *BMJ* have been women. None of the leading weekly general medical journals has yet been edited by a woman, but that day cannot be far off. Increasingly medical journals will employ women, and they may change the tone of the journals. To be modern and competitive journals need to make it easier for women to get on in the organisation, and providing child care facilities will be one element. Journals also need to be heard loudly and clearly in the debate over women in medicine.

The future of medicine

It's scary to be a young physician nowadays. You don't have to listen too hard to hear the grumblings of discontent among those in practice. Pessimism about the future abounds. Yet the reality for those of us who have trained long and hard is that, like it or not, we will need to work constructively within the present system. Our medical schools and training have done little to prepare us for these changes.[33]

David J Shulkin, MD, Pittsburgh

In the same issue of the *Journal of the American Medical Association* as that in which this quote appeared George Lundberg, the editor, wrote: 'In 1985, I published an editorial entitled "Medicine—A Profession in Trouble?" Unfortunately, in 1990 the question mark has come off.'[34] I left Britain in August 1989 with doctors deeply unhappy with the underfunding and hasty, untested reorganisation of the health service. I arrived in California to discover doctors even more unhappy. American doctors labour under the triple load of malpractice, bureaucratic and economic control of much of their work, and a health care system widely felt to be out of control. Worst of all, none of the players in the crisis in American health care seems to have the power to make an effective change.

Thus when I search the medical library at Stanford for articles on the future of medicine I find many but almost all of them have a despairing tone. Furthermore, they almost all talk about reorganising the delivery of care. It is rare to find a mention of the scientific developments that can be expected from the new biology. Doctors

197

seem to be too bogged down with the everyday miseries of trying to practise to pay much attention to possible scientific advances.

The despondent despairing tone of articles by doctors on the future of medicine contrasts noticeably with the upbeat optimistic tone of management articles on the future. Those graduating from business schools are raring to rip into the future, while medical students are profoundly wary. I do not believe that this need be so. The air of crisis that now affects both British and American doctors may be turned to advantage because it is out of crisis that profound organisational and cultural change can occur.[35]

The message of many of the articles on the future of medicine is that an age old professional tradition is being pillaged by business greed. These articles have, I believe, a rose tinted view of what professionalism means and an uninformed view of what management and business has to offer. After a year at business school I understand that business is less about junk bonds and leveraged buy outs and more about efficiency, effectiveness, team work, and quality—the very resources that medicine needs. Doctors and managers must, I believe, stop sniping at each other and start working together to offer the best and most cost effective health care that they can to everybody.

General medical journals have an important part to play in generating some confidence about the future. They must attempt to provide leadership through their editorial columns, ensure that their columns are open to a full range of informed opinion, bring new ideas to their readers, educate them on older ideas that have not reached doctors, and create some excitement around the possibilities of professional renewal.

DEVELOPMENTS IN MEDICAL SCIENCE

The two technologies that are blossoming and will drive medical developments in the next 10 to 20 years are computer technology and biotechnology. Both will have impacts through enabling medical research and through producing applications that can be used directly in health care. Furthermore, the two technologies are coming together. Naisbitt and Aburdene believe that the next decade will be the 'age of biology.'[2] 'Biology as a metaphor suggests information intensive, micro, inner adaptive, holistic.'

The 5000 volumes each of 1000 pages with 1000 words that is the human genome should be mapped and sequenced by the turn of the century, and that mapping will contribute to the understanding, diagnosis, and eventually treatment of not only single gene disorders

198

but also eventually polygenic disease. We are still, I think, decades away from the day when doctors will be able to read an embryo's genome, spot a defective gene, and replace it, but that day will surely be scientifically possible. Molecular biology will also in the next few decades make great progress with understanding cell differentiation, organ development, and chromosomal structure. It may be this work that will unlock effective treatments for cancer, and a deeper understanding of organogenesis may allow the growth of organs for transplantation and the regeneration of, for instance, dead heart muscle. This new biology also has the potential to increase hugely our understanding of the aging process.

Biotechnology will allow the production of many new proteins that may prove to have therapeutic potential. 'The body makes about 100 000 proteins,' says David Botstein, vice president for science at Genentech, the largest US biotechnology company. 'Suppose 1% of them have the potential to be turned into pharmaceuticals. That's 1000 new drugs.'[36] Or, equally upbeat: 'Genetic engineering will lead to the creation of a new age of vaccines,' says Kenneth Warren, formerly of the Rockefeller Foundation. 'It is almost inevitable that over the next 20 years it will become possible to produce vaccines through biotechnology for most infectious and parasitic causes of death.'[37] We should remember Ferkiss's discovery that scientists tend to be overoptimistic about the imminence and importance of scientific developments, but the new biology will produce rich rewards eventually—in understanding if nothing else.

Twenty years ago the first one kilobyte DRAM (dynamic random access memory) chip was created. Now four megabyte chips are in use. The power of computers is increasing exponentially, and this expansion combined with developments in software have meant that computers are being transformed from number crunchers into machines for insight and discovery. Computers like these will bring important advances in medical research—not least in neurosciences.

Supercomputers may also contribute to the replacement of randomised controlled trials with observational studies. Randomised controlled trials, although the crucial gold standard of treatment evaluation, are slow, expensive, and under attack from patients. They are, however, essential to produce comparable study groups and remove bias, but the power of the new computers may allow many more variables to be controlled out. Furthermore, once most hospital data (patient records, laboratory results, radiographic images, etc) are held on computer, supercomputers will be able to pose hypotheses and search the databases at night to test their hypotheses.

The other important development with computers will be that they will become much more user friendly. Doctors have not been able to harness the full power of computers because they are often uncomfortable with mathematics and keyboards, but the new computers will circumvent these problems. In addition, the computers will be tiny and fast, meaning that doctors will be able to make full use of them, and particularly of expert systems, in diagnosis and treatment. Computers will also be important in linking patients with support systems: thus computers will, for instance, read blood gas measurements and modify the ventilator as necessary.

But doctors need not worry that they will be put out of business by diseases being cured by a combination of biotechnology and computers. A poll of a group of doctors and medical researchers rated the probability of 'defeat of heart disease' by the year 2000 at 0·53, and they were more pessimistic about the 'defeat' of other conditions: AIDS (0·48), rheumatoid arthritis and multiple sclerosis (0·45), leukaemia and lung cancer (0·33), and Alzheimer's and Parkinson's diseases (0·15).[36]

Medical journals have been the primary traditional route for informing doctors of scientific developments, and they will undoubtedly continue this job. They must continue to apply strict scientific criteria to the publication of articles, but they may also need to develop doctors' scientific education. Many doctors are deeply ignorant about molecular biology, computer science, and other fast developing scientific subjects—and they must be helped to feel more comfortable with these subjects. Medical journals need to try to find a way to enthuse doctors with the intellectual excitement inherent in the subjects.

But in a broader sense medical journals need to keep science at the heart of the medical endeavour. A recent survey of the quality of medical evidence showed clearly the flimsiness of the scientific base of medicine.[38] This should not be taken as a signal to throw up our hands and keep on working by hunch but rather to redouble our efforts to make medicine more scientific while simultaneously keeping it human. Science and patient centred medicine are not incompatible.

THE FUTURE OF MEDICAL EDUCATION AND MEDICAL RESEARCH

The future of medicine clearly depends on excellent research and a continuing supply of well trained medical graduates. Both requirements are under threat in many countries. In both Britain and the US there are loud complaints about the small amount spent by governments on medical research. These complaints arise partly because research funds are no longer growing as fast as they did a decade ago, but also because the funds are being concentrated—meaning that those who are losing funds are squealing. This concentration will almost certainly continue, and the Institute for the Future is predicting that whereas the top 20 American medical schools account for 50% of all research funding in 1985 they will account for 56% by the year 2000.[39] The same process is happening and will continue to happen in Britain, where another trend is towards more directed research.

More of a threat to the future of medicine is the crisis in medical education. In Britain there is widespread unhappiness with the quality of medical education,[40] while in the US the number of applicants to medical school is falling, too many doctors are being produced,[41] and there is also widespread unhappiness with the quality of medical education.[42] One response in the US has been a widespread switch to problem based learning.[43] This trend will almost certainly continue and will spread increasingly to Britain. Medical education cannot be as dreary in the next decade as it was in the last.

Medical journals are intimately involved with medical education and research, and they must continue to pay attention not only to the output of the two activities but also to the process, commenting whenever possible with data and close argument rather than assertion.

THE FUTURE OF MEDICAL PRACTICE

Holism has become fashionable in the past few years and will, I believe, prove to be more than a fad. Indeed, I don't think that it ever was a fad. Although practitioners of alternative medicine have monopolised the term and implied that they were the first to practise it, the best orthodox doctors have always treated the whole patient. The Royal College of General Practitioners in Britain has long talked about tripartite diagnosis—meaning a physical, psychological, and social diagnosis—and the World Health Organisation long ago defined health as complete physical, mental, and social wellbeing. Some doctors may have been diverted for a while from holistic medicine as they succumbed to the idea that powerful technology alone could heal patients. Now even the most technologically

201

sophisticated practitioners recognise the importance of whole person medicine.

The notion of holism has a parallel in business—the recognition of how important it is to place the customer at the centre of your business. It is easy to pay lip service to such a notion but less easy to echo it throughout your organisation, but the most successful companies do it. The corollary in medicine will be to make patients the arbiters of outcome and quality. Elwood suggested in a far sighted Shattuck lecture in 1988 that a method of routinely surveying patients' quality of life be used as a way of linking together the currently competing interests of patients, payers, and providers.[44] 'In medicine,' he writes, 'we already have a consensus that our unifying goal is the good of the patient. To support this philosophy, I propose that we adopt a technology for collaborative action.'

One everyday reality that will accompany this return to putting patients at the centre of the medical endeavour will be a much better system of informed consent. Already, interactive videos have been developed that allow patients to inquire of other patients about the pluses and minuses of an operation like prostatectomy.

Another important development will be that quality in medical care will become a much more central issue—just as it has in manufacturing industry. About one in 20 hospital admissions results in an adverse event,[45] a proportion that seems far too high. Berwick has argued that doctors should study the (ironically, mostly American) techniques used by Japanese industry to open up a formidable quality gap and then apply them to health care.[46] This system, kaizen, does not descend on individuals; rather it uses statistical techniques to find ways continually to improve systems.[47] Such an approach has brought a rich return in manufacturing and should be able to do so in health care.

The concept of kaizen fits together with audit beacuse the process usually begins with a statistical study of what is happening at the moment—and often that study brings surprises. Quality assurance in the US has not been driven by doctors, but doctors in Britain have a chance to take the lead in auditing their practices and making improvements. The government has had to force the pace, but it seems thoroughly professional to measure what you do and try to improve on it, and doctors will surely be engaging much more in audit in a decade's time than they do at the moment. In recognition of this the *BMJ* started its monthly audit section at the beginning of 1990 and in 1992 the BMJ Publications Group will launch a new journal called *Quarterly Health Care*.

Medical practice will also in the next decade surely move further into preventive medicine. Once again this is an idea that has been voiced and supported for a long time, but it has been slow to happen. Patient pressure and legal consequences for those who neglect to take a patient's blood pressure will, however, force the pace.

Finally, medical practice will continue to move outside of hospitals. In the US this trend has been economically driven, but hospitals are increasingly recognised as being dangerous, unhealthy, infantilising places—and patients want to stay out of them as much as they can. Outpatient care and care by family doctors will continue to become more important.

General medical journals are the places where these issues will be debated and developed, and I believe that an increasing proportion of general journals will be devoted to these sorts of issues that are common and vital to the whole profession—and to the other members of the health team.

THE FUTURE OF PUBLIC HEALTH

Public health played a crucial role in the nineteenth and early twentieth centuries in reducing disease and extending life expectancy. Then its importance began to be forgotten as antibiotics and other effective forms of personal health care appeared. Now the central importance of public health care is being rediscovered, and the Institute of Medicine has recently defined the mission of public health—'to fulfill society's interest in assuring conditions in which people can be healthy'—and called for a resurgence in its power in the US.[48]

Medical journals have in recent years played an important part in the rediscovery of public health, and they must continue to press the profession and governments to give it the attention it needs.

THE FUTURE OF HEALTH CARE DELIVERY

It is the pressure to reform how health services are delivered that is most exercising doctors at the moment. Rogers, in his address to the New York Academy of Medicine on the future of medicine, said: 'To my sorrow, the major engine now driving change is the almost universal American perception that medical care is too expensive.'[49] In Britain an editorial in the *BMJ* has suggested that because of its current reorganisation 'the NHS is steaming ahead into an iceberg that will prove as devastating as the one that sank the Titanic.'[50] Everywhere, it seems, governments are concerned about overexpenditure on health care, while doctors are worried that they do not have enough resources to do their best by their patients. The gap between what could be done and can be afforded will continue to grow as populations age, technologies develop, and expectations expand.

Clearly no country has the answer about how to best provide cost effective health care to everybody, and countries will continue to experiment. It may be best then to think in very general terms about what the future may bring. Clearly societies cannot go on forever increasing the amount they spend on health care, and clearly there must be a point at which the return from any further expenditure on health care does not merit the expenditure. But where is that point? In markets for widgets that point is determined by how much consumers are willing to pay for the extra widget and how cheaply manufacturers can produce it. This system works so beautifully and efficiently for widgets, that advocates of the free market long to apply it to health care. Unfortunately it does not work for health care—largely because patients do not have enough information on outcome and cost to make economically sensible decisions; they also often do not know what they need and are not able, because of sickness, to make rational decisions. Furthermore, although it might be acceptable for somebody to be priced out of the market for widgets it's unacceptable (or should be) for parents to be priced out of the market for treating their child's leukaemia.[51]

These considerations rule out a free market in health care, but at the same time monopoly systems like the British National Health Service do not employ resources efficiently. Resources are allocated centrally and inevitably crudely, and decisions on expenditure are made by administrators and doctors without adequate information.[52]

Between these two poles there must be a better way, and the search is now on to find it. A better system (and there will be no perfect system) will depend on abundant information on costs and benefits and some sort of incentive to use resources in the most cost effective manner. Almost certainly the system will be funded from central taxation, and universal coverage will be essential. The experiments to move closer to such a system will continue into the next century, and surely both doctors and managers will want to cooperate in the attempt to find such a system. The skills and tools of both will be essential, and medical journals will be one of the main forums where the search is conducted. The primary contribution of medical journals will not be to lambast opponents and proponents of various ideas, but rather to ensure that the debate is conducted on as high a plane as possible with as many data and as much information as possible.

Included in this search for an equitable and efficient system will be technology assessment and detailed social discussions on what the benefits of health care are. Many of the tools needed for technology assessment are already available, but they are not as widely used as they should be.[53] Surely they will be used much more widely in the next decade, and medical journals should insist that they are. We want value not just effectiveness from new technology. Similarly, discussions among citizens on how to value the benefits of health care have already begun in Oregon,[54] and they will be seen much more widely. Medical journals should contribute to these discussions and make sure that their pages are not reserved for doctors alone.

The future of medical journals

I believe that the future for general medical journals—particularly those published in English—is bright. They will undoubtedly change, but they will not disappear. Electronic forms of publishing will become increasingly important after a hesitant start,[55] [56] but general journals will continue to exist in hard copy—not least because that is the comfortable way to read, particularly in the bath, but also because of the importance of serendipity in reading and learning.[57] Indeed, the buffeting and transforming of the medical profession over the next few decades will return general medical journals to their central function of gluing the profession together.

A few years ago there was much talk of the information explosion and an anxiety that we would be buried in information, if not knowledge and wisdom. But de Solla Price showed that this explosion was something of an illusion: publications had in fact been increasing at a constant 5–7% since the seventeenth century—in proportion with the number of scientists.[58] Since de Solla Price published his work the number of scientists has ceased to grow so fast—because of economic constraints—and the National Library of Medicine has been recording about 600 new medical journals annually during the past few years compared with about 1200 at the end of the '70s.[59]

The economics of libraries and journals are also playing a part in this slowing of the flood. Between 1977 and 1988 the average price of subscriptions to American journals within the US increased from $51 to $180, and the rise in the price of journals has consistently run ahead of inflation. These trends have led one of the librarians at the New York Academy of Medicine to predict that 'unless librarians and academicians devise a long-term solution to the cost problem, they [medical libraries] may [by the year 2000] resemble little more than bookstores containing random and sporadic bits of information.'[58]

The trend described by de Solla Price was for general journals to beget specialist journals, which then beget superspecialist journals and so on until we have about five tiers. The same trend leads general journals to shift from original papers, which will be appreciated by only a few readers, to review articles, which appeal to many. Already the editors of general journals are faced with the paradox that much of the effort of editors and subeditors goes into the part of the journal—the original articles—that are least read. Would not it be sensible then, asks the disinterested reader, for general journals to abandon original papers and concentrate on reviews and other general material? But down that road lies, I believe, disaster. The important general journals are set apart from the many review journals and medical newspapers by the fact that they do publish original papers. Sometimes these original papers are of large general importance, and even when they are not they serve to remind editors and readers that science is at the heart of the best general medical journals.

But general medical journals will become increasingly general, with more news, comment, correspondence, and educational material. They will contain more material on health policy, and they will become increasingly international. I think that these trends are already apparent in the *BMJ*. Meanwhile, the first tier of specialist journals—for instance, those for paediatricians—will also become more general. These journals will also continue to exist in hard copy, whereas the superspecialist journals may eventually appear primarily in electronic form.

The increasing professionalisation of medical journals, with higher standards of peer review, guidelines on statistics and the like, rules on dual publication, and limits on the number of authors will undoubtedly continue, but I do not foresee a college of medical editing with a president and an exam. Medical editors enjoy the roguish aspects of journalism, and an element of adolescent iconoclasm is, I believe, useful to editors. It may also be that some of the proliferation of peer review will be rolled back if it reaches the point where it is bureacratically too heavy and too prone to stifling the creative and innovative.[60] [61]

Electronic databases, full text retrieval services for some journals, and a few electronic journals are already here, but many doctors have little or no interaction with electronic forms of publishing. There will, I think, be steady but unspectacular developments in electronic publishing. Firstly, general journals may use electronic publishing as a sort of supplement for providing interested readers with extensive data and for publishing negative results. Secondly, superspecialist journals will 'fade to electronic' either on line or on CD–ROMs. Thirdly, journals will increasingly be available in electronic form as well as continuing to be in hard copy. I did some of the research for this paper on a machine in the Stanford Business School which searches for and provides abstracts of hundreds of current business publications; in addition, it will provide from a laser printer a facsimile version of some of the papers. The fascimiles are stored on CD-ROMs. No equivalent exists for medicine, but the extraordinary popularity of this machine seems to suggest that it represents one part of the future. Fourthly, interactive CD–ROMs like the one produced on AIDS will become increasingly important: sophisticated software will allow doctors to ask questions of their 'journals.' Electronic forms of publishing may become more important in developing countries if the price of hardware continues to fall dramatically but, failing that, publication on microfiche and free dissemination to developing countries will continue to be crucial.

Electronic information will also become more important for editors. Most of the *BMJ* editors now write on computers, and an office computer tracks manuscripts through the office and keeps records of referees. But little editing is done on the screen, few papers are received electronically, and the editors are not regularly searching databases. All of these things will, I think, become much more common over the next decade as a new generation of doctors familiar with computers passes through, as computers become more user friendly, and as databases become larger, more useful, and more accessible.[62] One thing that will be particularly important will be searching databases to try to reduce plagiarism, fraud, and dual publication.

Conclusion

The approach of the millennium is causing great excitement among soothsayers and futurologists, and the feeling that something important is afoot is increased by the dramatic changes in eastern Europe and South Africa. For sure the world will be very different in 10 years' time, and this may be more true for doctors than some other parts of the population. Change can be terrifying, but it also can be invigorating and exciting. I hope that medical journals can capture a spirit of excitement as their world changes. After all, they are not far removed from newspapers, and change is news. My last prediction—made with confidence—is that life will not be dull in the next few decades.

1 Pile S. *The return of heroic failures*. Harmondsworth, Middlesex: Penguin, 1989.
2 Naisbett J, Aburdene P. *Megatrends 2000: ten new directions for the 1990s*. New York: Morrow, 1990.
3 *Future Medical Almanac*.
4 Porter ME. *Competitive strategy: techniques for analysing industries and competitors*. New York: Free Press, 1980.
5 Porter ME. *Competitive advantage: creating and sustaining superior performance*. New York: Free Press, 1985.
6 Peters TJ, Waterman RH. *In search of excellence: lessons from America's best run companies*. New York: Warner Books, 1983.
7 Porter ME. *The competitive advantage of nations*. New York: Free Press, 1990.
8 Amara R. A note on what we have learned about the methods of futures planning. *Technological Forecasting and Social Change* 1989;**36**:43–7.
9 Ehrlich PR, Ehrlich AH. *The population explosion*. New York: Simon and Schuster, 1990.
10 Worldwatch Institute. *State of the world*. New York: W W Norton, 1990.
11 Bellamy E. *Looking backward 2000–1887*. New York: Ticknor, 1887.
12 Osborn F. *Our plundered planet*. Boston: Little, Brown, 1948.
13 Orwell G. *Nineteen eighty-four*. London: Secker and Warburg, 1949.
14 Meadows D, Meadows DL, Randers J, Behrens WW III. *The limits to growth*. New York: Universe Books, 1972.
15 Huxley A. *Brave new world*. New York: Doubleday, 1932.
16 Huxley A. *Island*. London: Chatto and Windus, 1975.
17 Ferkiss VC. *Futurology: promise, performance, prospects. The Washington papers*. Vol 5. Beverly Hills: Sage Publications, 1977.
18 Kahn H, Weiner AJ. *The year 2000*. New York: Macmillan, 1967.
19 Bell D. *The coming of postindustrial society. A venture in social forecasting*. New York: Basic Books, 1976.
20 Wall Street Journal. *Here comes tomorrow*. Princeton: Dow Jones, 1967.
21 Institute for the Future. *1990 ten year forecast*. Menlo Park, California: Institute for the Future, 1990.
22 Anonymous. This year's model. *Economist* 1990;May 26:93–4.
23 Anonymous. *Saving the ozone layer: London conference*. London: Central Office of Information, 1989.
24 Gray M, Keeble B. Greening the NHS [editorial]. *Br Med J* 1989;**299**:4.
25 McKie RM, Rycroft MJ. Health and the ozone layer [editorial]. *Br Med J* 1988;**297**:369.
26 Bach GL, Flanagan R, Howell J, Levy F, Lima A. *Microeconomics*. Englewood Cliffs, New Jersey: Prentice-Hall, 1987.
27 Robock SH, Simmonds K. *International business and multinational enterprises*. Homewood, Illinois: Irwin, 1989.
28 Pechter J. Workplace openers. In: Wall Street Journal. *Workplace of the future*. Wall Street Journal Reports. New York: Dow Jones, 1990.
29 Drucker PF. The coming of the new organization. *Harvard Business Review* 1988;**66**:4553.

30 Wall Street Journal. *Workplace of the future*. Wall Street Journal Reports. New York: Dow Jones, 1990.
31 Tushman M, Nadsler D. Organising for innovation. *California Management Review* 1986;**28**:74–92.
32 Schwartz FN. Management women and the new facts of life. *Harvard Business Review* 1989;**67**:65–76.
33 Shulkin DJ. Cost effectiveness and the future of medicine. *JAMA* 1990;**263**:40.
34 Lundberg GD. Countdown to millennium—balancing the professionalism and business of medicine. *JAMA* 1990;**263**:86.
35 Pascale RT. *Managing on the edge*. New York: Simon and Schuster, 1990.
36 Bylinsky G. Technology in the year 2000. *Fortune* 1988; July 18:92–8.
37 Warren K. Quoted in: Naisbett J, Aburdene P. *Megatrends 2000: ten new directions for the 1990s*. New York: Morrow, 1990.
38 Eddy DM, Billings J. The quality of medical evidence: implications for quality of care. *Health Aff (Millwood)* 1988 Spring;**7**:19–32.
39 Amara R, Morrison JI, Schmid G. *Looking ahead at American health care*. Washington: McGraw-Hill, 1988.
40 Smith R. Medical education and the GMC: controlled or stifled? *Br Med J* 1989;**298**:1372–5.
41 Tarlov AR. How many physicians is enough? *JAMA* 1990;**263**:571–2.
42 Kay J. Traumatic deidealisation and the future of medicine. *JAMA* 1990;**263**:572–3.
43 Barrows HS, Tamblyn R. *Problem based learning*. New York: Springer-Verag, 1980.
44 Ellwood PM. Shattuck lecture—outcomes management. A technology of patient experience. *N Engl J Med* 1988;**318**:1549–56.
45 Harvard Medical Practice Study. *Patients, doctors, and lawyers: medical injury, malpractice litigation, and patient compensation in New York*. Cambridge, Massachusetts: Harvard Medical Practice Study, 1990.
46 Berwick DM. Continuous improvement as an ideal in health care. *N Eng J Med* 1989;**320**:53–6.
47 Imai M. *Kaizen: the key to Japan's competitive success*. New York: McGraw Hill, 1986.
48 Institute of Medicine. *The future of public health*. Washington DC, National Academy Press, 1988.
49 Rogers DE. Thoughts on the future of medicine. *Bull N Y Acad Med* 1989;**65**:859–65.
50 Smith T. Politicians and scientists. *BMJ* 1990;**300**:1283–4.
51 Morrison I. In: Institute for the Future. *1990 ten year forecast*. Menlo Park, California: Institute for the Future, 1990.
52 Enthoven AC. *Reflections on the management of the National Health Service*. London: Nuffield Provincial Hospitals Trust, 1985.
53 Institute of Medicine. *Assessing medical technologies*. Washington: Institute of Medicine, 1985.
54 Egan T. Oregon lists illnesses by priority to see who gets Medicaid care. *New York Times* 1990 January: A1, A18.
55 Gurndsey J. *Electronic publishing trends in the United States and Europe*. Oxford: Learned Information, 1982.
56 British Library. *Electronic publishing and the UK*. London: British Library, 1986.
57 Relman AS. Anniversary discourse: the purposes and prospects of the general medical journal. *Bull N Y Acad Med* 1988;**64**:875–80.
58 de Solla Price D. *Science since Babylon*. New Haven: Yale University Press, 1961.
59 Pascarelli AM. Guest editorial: will libraries exist in the year 2000? The effect of prices on collections. *Bull N Y Acad Med* 1989;**65**:859–65.
60 Smith R. Problems with peer review and alternatives. *Br Med J* 1988;**296**:774–7.

61 Roy R. Peer review of proposals—rationale, practice, and performance. *Bulletin of Science and Technology in Society* 1982;**2**:405–22.
62 Smith R. One man's electronic fantasy. *Med J Aust* 1987;**146**:589 and 592.

Index

217